Nursing Care
of the
Older Person

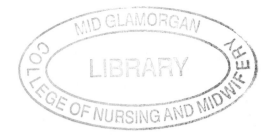

Nursing Care
of the
Older Person

Jane Farrell, R.N., B.S.
Former Nursing Instructor and
Educator in Senior Services
Bellin Memorial Hospital
Green Bay, Wisconsin

J. B. Lippincott   Philadelphia
Grand Rapids   New York   St. Louis   San Francisco
London   Sydney   Tokyo

Acquisitions Editor: Patricia L. Cleary
Coordinating Editorial Assistant: Nancy Lyons
Manuscript Editor: Dorothy Wright
Indexer: Victoria Boyle
Art Director: Susan Blaker
Cover Photo: Barbara Proud
Production Manager: Carol A. Florence
Production Editor: Kathy Crown
Production Coordinator: Kathryn Rule
Compositor: Digitype, Inc.
Text Printer/Binder: R.R. Donnelly & Sons
Cover Printer: Algen Press

3 5 6 4 2

Library of Congress Cataloging-in-Publication Data

Farrell, Jane.
  Nursing care of the older person / Jane Farrell.
     p.   cm.
  Includes bibliographies and index.
  ISBN 0-397-54738-2
  1. Geriatric nursing,   I. Title.
  [DNLM: 1. Aging.   2. Geriatric Nursing.   WY 152 F245n]
PC954.F37   1990
610.73'65 — dc20
DNLM/DLC
for Library of Congress   89-12662
                                                                          CIP

Any procedure or practice described in this book should be applied by the health-care practitioner under appropriate supervision in accordance with professional standards of care used with regard to the unique circumstances that apply in each practice situation. Care has been taken to confirm the accuracy of information presented and to describe generally accepted practices. However, the author, editors, and publisher cannot accept any responsibility for errors or omissions or for consequences from application of the information in this book and make no warranty, express or implied, with respect to the contents of the book.

Every effort has been made to ensure drug selections and dosages are in accordance with current recommendations and practice. Because of ongoing research, changes in government regulations and the constant flow of information on drug therapy, reactions and interactions, the reader is cautioned to check the package insert for each drug for indications, dosages, warnings, and precautions, particularly if the drug is new or infrequently used.

10.12.92

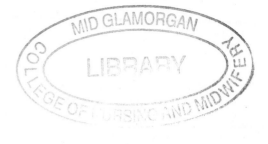

To my husband, Mike,
with whom I am growing
older . . . quite easily,
in mutual love and respect.

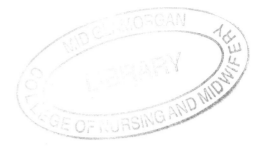

Preface

This book introduces the nursing student to the various aspects of caring for, and *about*, older people. A brief history of aging in our society with a perspective on the present and future is included because the characteristics of the older population, societal attitudes and feelings, and the trends and issues of aging have implications for nursing. A review of the development of geriatric nursing and how the nursing process works in this field provides background material and reference points. Throughout the book I have strived to emphasize the individuality of the older person in sickness and wellness. For this reason, communication is both a separate chapter and discussed frequently in the text. Common problems of aging are described in Chapter 6, with suggestions for nursing care in the hospital or nursing home and suggestions for family teaching. Content about nursing care focuses on the prevention, diagnosis, and solving of problems, on providing comfort, and on setting realistic goals. I hope this will help the nursing student to identify and meet basic needs, rather than concentrating on, for example, a "cardiac patient."

Some exploration of personal philosophy is suggested as the student is asked to consider aging persons and patients as role models. My daughter once said, "No one will talk to me about what it's like to be old. I got advice on how to get through puberty, how to be a teenager, and how to get through college. I never asked for any of it. But nobody will tell me about getting old." I hope this book will offer some insights about growing old that will enrich the understanding of the aging process for each nursing student or nurse who reads it.

JANE FARRELL, R.N., B.S.

Acknowledgements

As I wrote this book there was scarcely anyone around me who was not aware of it! I marvel at the patience and willingness of family, friends, casual acquaintances, and strangers who made completion of this project a reality. To acknowledge all of them individually is impossible.

I will say a special "thank you" to Tom Arndt, president of Bellin Hospital, for providing me with the facilities and services I needed to write this book. At Bellin I had moral, physical, and mental support whenever I needed it, and from whomever I asked. The following people from my Bellin life must also be thanked because they were part of the process from the very beginning and remained with me to the end: George Kerwin, Senior Vice President; Kay Schaus, R.N., Discharge Planner; Vonnie Verkuilen, R.N., College of Nursing; and the staff of Two North. Cindy Reinl and her staff in the Health Sciences Library, particularly Melody Robb, were exceptionally helpful.

Barb Long, R.N., Director of Nursing at the Grancare Nursing Center, was a constant assistant. Resource people throughout the year included Avice Kerr, R.N.; Elaine Johnson, retired teacher; Dr. and Mrs. John Ryder, retired dentist and his wife; Eunice Schrevens, dancer; and Fred H. Walbrun, M.D.

Family members, and professional and personal friends posed for my pictures, as did gracious strangers. Shirley Farrell and my husband, Mike, took the photographs. There were those who helped my assistant and daughter, Sheila, through her computer woes.

I am deeply grateful to Gray Panther Maggie Kuhn, singer and lecturer Pearl Bailey, and Sister Pam Moehring at Mount Mary College, Milwaukee, as the first correspondents to offer encouragement and help.

Support for this project from the following community resources is gratefully acknowledged: University Bank, Beltone Hearing Service, Streu's Pharmacy, Grancare Nursing Center, Americana Healthcare Center, Brown County Commission on Aging, Senior Citizens Center,

Bellin Health Connection, and Cedar Creek Adult Care Home. I acknowledge the assistance and support of Julie Guilette.

I would like to thank my editor, Patricia L. Cleary, and her assistant, Nancy Lyons, for their guidance and good will. Patti's sense of humor and calm reassurance were friendly and therapeutic.

To all of these people, and to everyone else who wandered smiling and helpful into my life this past year, I say from my heart, thank you and God bless.

Contents

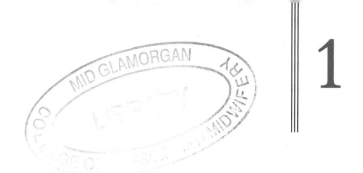

1

Aging: Past, Present, and Future

Learning Objectives

When you complete this chapter, you should be able to:

1. *Give examples of how older people were or were not valued throughout history.*
2. *List three reasons why society is aging.*
3. *Describe how today's elderly have witnessed the 20th century.*
4. *Define, with examples, the term "ageism."*
5. *Discuss truths about aging and older people.*
6. *Explain why a nurse should remain informed about trends that affect the aging population.*
7. *Discuss nursing roles and the major issues in aging.*
8. *Give an example of how a nurse becomes involved in ethical issues.*

My grandpa went out walking
In his sneakers in the snow.
It mattered not how cold it was,
Or where he meant to go.
He didn't believe in doctors,
Always had a better way.
He mixed and matched home remedies
While the rest of us would pray.
He did exactly as he pleased.
There was nothing we could do.
It's tough to win an argument
With a man who's eighty-two.

—J.F.

Life at any age can be rewarding, yet most of us resist the thought of growing older. Why is this? Although aging is not always pleasant, it is a natural process we will all experience. A reluctance to age is based partly on common myths, or falsehoods, about what older people are like.

Our world can be a difficult place in which to grow old. Then, too, the thought of getting old is associated with thoughts about dying. For those who do not acknowledge death as part of their own lives, aging is unacceptable. Confronting and dealing with these attitudes and feelings does not mean one has to like getting old, but it does permit a better understanding of the changes that will occur as one ages.

Current population statistics show that attitudes about aging and the aged are changing. Trends in providing and financing health care, for instance, reflect a growing concern for the needs of older people. Issues that affect quality of life are receiving more attention.

Aging in the Past

Prehistoric and Ancient

As far back as prehistoric times, chronological old age was virtually unknown. A life much past the age of 40 was remarkable. In primitive societies, discrepancies existed between legends and life-styles. Sacred myths represented many gods as wise and ancient men and credited old women with protecting hunters and fishermen. In reality, when aged people hindered movement or were a drain on the resources of the group, they were abandoned or encouraged to wander off by themselves.

In ancient China, the teachings of Confucius placed the entire household under the authority of the family's oldest living man. Women were oppressed until they became old, and they then assumed control of all the children. "Honor thy father and mother" was the commandment given to Moses in the Old Testament.

Greek and Roman poets and philosophers puzzled over the riches of old age as opposed to the joys of being young. We find aging heroes, both wise *and* foolish, in the works of Shakespeare and others.

An American History of Aging and Attitudes

In the days of Pilgrims and Puritans, and the struggle to settle the eastern seaboard, few people lived to see old age. When they did, they were highly respected. To age was to overcome death, so senior citizens were heroes. No one was considered "over the hill" in colonial America. Men of age, because they had weathered the storms of life and become, supposedly, moderate and wise, were preferred in colonial politics. Young colonial Americans wanted to look older, and some wore white wigs in an effort to conceal their youth. Clothes were designed to be just as concealing; men's coats had narrow, rounded shoulders, and britches were broad in the hip and waist.

A family's land was the measure of its wealth. The father usually held on to it, well into his old age, while his sons worked the land for him. The youth of colonial America obeyed their elders.

Attitudes changed with growth of the new nation. The expansion of the frontier brought opportunities for the young to leave father and home. Pioneers in the wilderness became the new American heroes. The growth of cities and the rise of industry created a larger job market, making it possible for young people to build lives independent of their families, to accumulate wealth, and to gain power and prestige. Youth became the time of life for recognition through personal accomplishment.

The authors and poets of the United States, like those in Europe had done for centuries, both lamented and praised the aged and aging. Was old age a gift, a curse, or both? Ralph Waldo Emerson wrote, "We do not count a man's years until he has nothing else to count." Longfellow wrote, "For age is opportunity and no less . . . Than youth itself . . ."

Today's Older Population

Our older population is classified as follows:

Young-old: 65–74 years of age
Middle-old: 75–84 years of age
Old-old: 85+ years of age

Although each group has had a different experience, all of our older population has been affected by the sweeping changes of the 20th century.

Between 1900 and 1920, the world acquired the airplane, submarine, radio, and Einstein's theory of relativity, and was permanently changed by the events of World War I. About 14 million immigrants arrived on this nation's shores full of vitality and dreams. The children they had and the children they brought with them are among today's elderly. They grew up when the childhood diseases of smallpox, scarlet fever, diphtheria, and whooping cough, along with other infections and diseases, were claiming many lives. Research into the prevention of communicable diseases was growing. Labor laws were enacted. In 1920, women gained the right to vote.

While only a few of them were old enough to fight in "the war to end all wars" — World War I — the majority of our now-elderly citizens produced the sons, grandsons, and great grandsons who would fight in World War II, the Korean War, and the Vietnam War.

The great depression that followed the stock market crash of 1929 was a grim reality for this age group. Raising families was a major challenge, and it left many of today's old people with the fear that they could go hungry again and with the belief that wasting food is a sin.

Americans who are 65 to 75 years of age were children or teenagers during the great depression. The benefits of vaccination, immunization, the sulfonamides and penicillin would belong to them and their families. Automobiles and airplanes would broaden their horizons. Having known how hard life could be, more and more of them saw the value of education and would impress that upon their own children.

Poliomyelitis — "polio" — or infantile paralysis was a dreaded disease that most commonly struck children. The first epidemic occurred in 1942, and with succeeding epidemics polio killed or paralyzed large numbers of Americans until Jonas Salk developed a vaccine in 1954.

The veterans of World War II were left with a deep patriotism that often caused them to endorse loyally their nation's military and defense commitments. In later years, this patriotism became a wedge between older and younger generations. The societal upheaval during the Vietnam War is a striking example of that generational conflict. The assassinations in the 1960s of President John Kennedy, Robert Kennedy, and Martin Luther King remain vivid and shocking memories for today's older population.

From childhood to old age, our very oldest population experienced and observed tremendous technological advances and lived through extremes. They can recollect the horse and buggy while watching space flight on television. The elderly citizens of today were witness to the 20th century.

Aging in the Present

Myths and Truths

The physical changes of aging that we observe in many older adults show us the limitations and deficits of growing old. Aging people do not always see well, hear well, or move around easily. Aches and pains are common, and some have problems with short-term memory. All of this contributes to myths and falsehoods about aging. Separating the myths of aging from the truths is a first step in understanding one's own feelings and in forming positive attitudes about older people.

Myth: Old Age is a Disease

The truth is that growing old is a normal physiological process, the end stage of life called "senescence." Old age is linked with disease for various reasons. One reason is that 65% of all older adults have at least one chronic but not necessarily disabling disease. Another is that immunity lessens with age, so older people are more susceptible to infections. Potential problems of aging, such as stiffness and tremors, are often mistaken by others as signs of disease. Also, since people tend to discuss things they have in common, it often appears to others that older people "always" talk about their illnesses. Therefore, it is assumed that all old persons are ill. The truth is that about 95% of all aging adults live independently or with minimal assistance and are in reasonably good health.

Myth: Old Age Begins at 65

Why should it? There is no biological switch in the human body that automatically switches to "decline" on a person's 65th birthday.

Chancellor von Bismarck of Germany should receive the credit or the blame for the choice of 65 years as a marker of old age. In the 1880s, Bismarck settled on this age as the best age to retire his military personnel.

The truth is that most Americans do not retire at the age of 65. Individual Retirement Accounts (IRAs) have made it possible for many people to retire after they are 59, and it is becoming a common practice in the business world to provide incentives to employees to retire before 65. On the other end of the scale, federal legislation in 1978 raised the mandatory retirement age to 70. Older Americans now have some choice in the matter.

Today, if one wished to choose a marker for the onset of old age, it would be necessary to consider the continuing rise in life expectancy. Then, perhaps, 75 or even 80 years of age would be a more appropriate marker.

The human organism begins to age at conception, since growth is aging. Each person ages individually throughout a lifetime because of different genetics, self-care, life-style, and chance. Certainly, one's outlook and ability to adjust to changes that occur with time are additional factors.

Myth: Old Age Brings Senility

Senility is a catchall term meaning "state of mental deterioration." Senility is not due to old age. The majority of Americans over age 65 show no signs of mental decline. Normal aging results in short-term memory loss and delayed reaction time. Both conditions produce behaviors that seem to indicate mental impairment. Loss of hearing and lack of motivation often make older people appear dull. The truth is that there is no loss of intelligence or creativity as one grows older (Fig. 1–1). In fact, there are numerous examples of people becoming more creative with age. Michelangelo began his architectural work on St. Peter's Cathedral in Rome when he was 71. Comedian and actor George Burns became *more* well known in his 90s, and folk artist Grandma Moses first gained recognition at 78 (see "Senior Superstars" display).

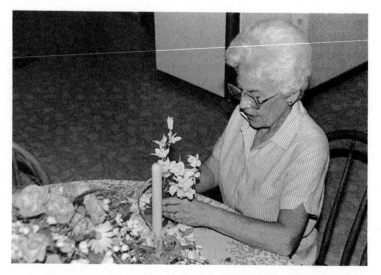

Figure 1–1. Many older people are creative in arts and crafts.

Senior Superstars

VOLTAIRE—One of the greatest 18th century European authors, he wrote his best works, including *Candide*, after the age of 64

BENJAMIN FRANKLIN—A framer of the Constitution at age 81

VERDI—Italian composer, wrote his opera, *Falstaff*, at age 80

WILLIAM HARVEY—English physician, described circulation of the blood and defined the heart as a pump when he was 73

DISRAELI—Prime Minister of Great Britain for the second time, at the age of 70

GOLDA MEIR—At age 71, she became Prime Minister of Israel

HENRY FORD—Introduced the V-8 engine at age 69

CLAUDE PEPPER—A Democratic Congressman from Florida in his 80s; he advocated rights for senior citizens.

JAMES MICHENER—Author of *Tales of the South Pacific* and many other books, writing into his 80s

SOHN KEE CHUNG—At age 76, carried the Olympic torch in the 1988 summer games; he is still a runner, and Korea's greatest marathoner

NELSON MANDELA—Black nationalist, at age 70, serving life imprisonment for his political activities

MARY MARTIN—Became the world's favorite Peter Pan on stage at age 40, returned to the stage at age 72

MAGGIE KUHN—Founded the Gray Panthers, a political organization for older people, after her retirement; she describes two advantages of being in her 80s: outliving her opposition and being able to speak her mind.

Myth: Older People are Very Much Alike

Norms of behavior are easy to establish for newborns and young children. A few generalizations can be made about adolescents and young adults. As we get older we get less and less alike, so that by the time we are middle-aged, comparison becomes difficult, and at 70 it is impossible. There is no such creature as an "average" old person.

The improved health status of older people calls attention to their individuality. In institutional settings, sick and dependent people in their 70s are being cared for by healthy, energetic women and men who are nursing personnel or volunteers also in their 70s. It is not unusual to hear about people in their 70s who are still in top physical and mental condition and are directing large corporations.

Likes and dislikes, interests, and abilities in the older age groups are diverse. Social and economic circumstances contribute to the differences among them. The myth that older people are all alike may have led us to believe that at a certain age a person cannot make decisions about how to spend leisure time. This accounts for the false notion that all older adults want to be called "senior citizens" and herded into group activities. The truth is that with adequate finances and available family and friends, older people, like the rest of us, choose activities that suit their preferences (Fig. 1 – 2).

Myth: Older People are Usually Unhappy

Life satisfaction has little to do with age. Optimism, which contributes to happiness, is not a quality limited to the young. We tend to confuse the desire to be young with unhappiness. If an older person says, "I'd give anything to be your age again," it does not necessarily mean he or she is unhappy. It is a rare person who would not appreciate the chance to repeat some aspect of his lifetime. Old people who are chronically unhappy may have always been that way. Personality change is not part of the aging process but is an individual development. We take our personalities into old age with us.

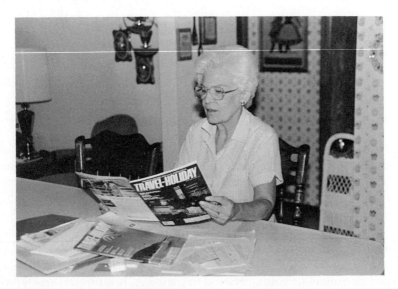

Figure 1 – 2. Older people often have the time and money to try new adventures.

Myth: Older People are Set in Their Ways and Unable to Change

Some attitudes and habits become fixed as one grows older. Often these are the things that work for a person. The church that "feels right," the doctor whom one has learned to trust, the political viewpoints that are compatible, and the daily routines that are comfortable — these are some examples of set ways. The truth is that old age brings major socioeconomic changes to which a person must and does adapt, such as selling a home and moving, living alone, and living on a fixed income.

Myth: Older People are Sexless

Hormonal and tissue changes that occur with aging may diminish sexual capacity, but age has little to do with sexual drive and dreams. Sexuality means more than the ability to have intercourse; it includes love, warmth, touch, and intimacy. The truth is that the need to share and express sexuality is lifelong.

Myth: In General, Older People are Lonely and Socially Isolated

Old people are not usually abandoned, although our attention is caught by accounts in newspapers and television of those who are. Studies suggest that the majority of older adults have close relatives and friends and are busy with activities and organizations (Fig. 1–3). The truth is that as they grow older many people find they have time to do those things they never had time for when they were young.

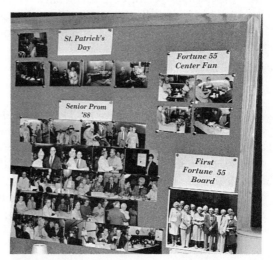

Figure 1–3. Older people are not usually lonely or socially isolated.

Myth: People Become More Religious as They Age

In many cases it seems that they do. Yet it is often true that the older person has become, with age, less concerned about what people think of him and his viewpoints. Life's crises have more influence than age on the development of spirituality and commitment to a particular church. The loss of a loved one may cause an individual to seek consolation and answers in religious faith. Grandma may simply have more time to read her Bible now than she did when she was younger. Another truth is that many older people who are religious were religious when they were younger.

Myth: Most Older Workers Cannot Work as Effectively as Younger Workers

Actually, older workers are not only good workers, but they have fewer accidents than younger workers. They also tend to have more stable lives and fewer outside commitments, so they are more flexible about the hours they can work. Absenteeism due to illness is not a problem among older employees. An older person is also more apt to be contented in a job.

Myth: Most Old People are Poor

While Social Security is hardly a windfall, it has reduced the number of poor elderly. The January, 1988 issue of *AARP News Bulletin*, from the American Association of Retired Persons, reported that one out of every five older persons is living just above or below the poverty level. It is true that many older persons are financially well off, and one estimate is that more than a half million persons 65 or older are millionaires. In addition, most of the money in savings and loan institutions belongs to people over 55 years of age.

Myth: Older People Have no Power

In 1935, President Franklin D. Roosevelt signed the Social Security Act, which established a system in which people over 65 can be assured of retirement benefits. Since then, older Americans have become increasingly active in making their needs known and in influencing political and social groups. The First National Conference on Aging, in 1950, was the beginning of a steady stream of developments on behalf of older people. The chart, "Milestones for Senior Citizens," highlights legislation and other actions.

1951—Federal Committee on Aging created to coordinate programs for the aging

1956—US Department of Health, Education and Welfare establishes a special staff on aging, which evolves into the Office of Aging

1959—A Senate subcommittee begins to consider problems of aging and the aged; Federal Council on Aging established at Cabinet level

1960—First appropriation authorizing direct loans for housing for the elderly, from Housing Act of 1959

1961—First White House Conference on Aging produces the Senior Citizen's Charter or Bill of Rights

1962—President's Council on Aging replaces Federal Council

1963—President John F. Kennedy designates May as Senior Citizens Month

1965—President Lyndon B. Johnson signs Older Americans Act, which deals with older people's income, health, housing, social, and legal needs; Foster Grandparent Program initiated; Medicare established

1967—Age Discrimination in Employment Act ended discrimination against people 40–65 years of age

1971—Second White House Conference on Aging

1972—Supplemental Security Program for the Aged to provide minimal income

1975—House of Representatives Special Committee on Aging

1978—Federal legislation banned mandatory retirement for many workers under age 70

1980—National Hispanic Council on Aging established to address needs of older Hispanics; development of educational materials is an ongoing function

1981—Third White House Conference on Aging—Growing needs of the elderly were recognized in the areas of health, housing, and minimum income; the need to safeguard Social Security is addressed

1983—Diagnostic Related Groups (DRGs) created to control Medicare costs

1986—Congress passes legislation to establish ten Alzheimer's Disease treatment centers throughout country; bill was sponsored by Congressman Claude Pepper

1988—Retirement Income and Employment Subcommittee of the Select Committee on Aging working on S.S.I. reform to bring benefits up to poverty level, among other things

Professional and voluntary organizations have responded to the needs of older Americans in various ways. The American Geriatrics Society, founded in 1942, and the Gerontological Society, Inc., established in 1944, were two of the earliest groups to recognize the unique needs of the elderly, and their journals are still being published.

The American Medical Association organized a Committee on Aging in 1955. In 1954, the Senior Citizens of America was organized, with the American Society for the Aged, Inc., close behind it in 1955. As the fastest growing population in the country, the elderly have a great deal of power and the potential for even more (see the "Senior Citizens Charter" display).

"Ageism" is discrimination against individuals as they grow older. Public awareness of such discrimination in our society is growing, but ageism is still prevalent.

Today's world was designed for youthful bodies and capabilities. For older citizens, visits to public bathrooms, riding elevators, and entering or exiting buildings, can be hazardous trips. Too many signs have small or otherwise unreadable messages. Stairways are narrow and high, and hall-ways are darkened. The steps into most buses are perilous to climb. An older person with any degree of limited motion can hardly cross a street before the traffic light changes.

Once a person reaches middle-age, society does not even allow him to fully enjoy his birthday. The man who chooses to regard his 50th birth-day as a positive event is soon reminded, by a comic card from a friend, that it is not a joyous occasion at all.

In 1979, Pat Moore, 26 years old, disguised herself and became an 85-year-old woman for one day each week for three years. Working in the field of industrial design, she had observed that the limitations of older citizens were not taken into account by industry, for instance, in the design of an automobile. To expand her knowledge of older people and how their needs could be addressed in her field, she decided to expe-rience their problems and feelings. In her book, *Disguised*, she tells how she was treated on the streets and in parks all over North America, as the characters she portrayed. At various times she was a rich old woman, a woman of moderate means, or a bag lady. While she met many caring and gentle people, her book is an eye-opener about discrimination. As an old woman—and especially as a poor old woman—she was ignored, pushed, and cheated. Her worst experience was being beaten and robbed in Harlem, which left one of her hands with nerve damage. Her book is a testimony to the ways in which society has made victims of old people.

Ageism has resulted in some older persons becoming passive, resigned members of society, with low self-esteem. The great tragedy in this is the waste of knowledge, ability, and talent.

Senior Citizen's Charter

Each of our Senior Citizens, regardless of race, color or creed, is entitled to:

The right to be useful.
The right to obtain employment, based on merit.
The right to freedom from want in old age.
The right to a fair share of the community's recreational, educational, and medical resources.
The right to obtain decent housing suited to needs of later years.
The right to the moral and financial support of one's family so far as is consistent with the best interest of the family.
The right to live independently, as one chooses.
The right to live and die with dignity.
The right of access to all knowledge as available on how to improve the later years of life.

Balancing these rights are:

The obligation of each citizen to prepare himself to become and resolve to remain active, alert, capable, self-supporting and useful so long as health and circumstances permit and to plan for ultimate retirement.
The obligation to learn and apply sound principles of physical and mental health.
The obligation to seek and develop potential avenues of service in the years after retirement.
The obligation to make available the benefits of his experience and knowledge.
The obligation to endeavor to make himself adaptable to the changes added years will bring.
The obligation to attempt to maintain such relationships with family, neighbors and friends as will make him a respected and valued counselor throughout his later years.

Established by the first White House Conference on Aging, 1961.

The impact of ageism on younger or middle-aged people is that they usually prefer to discuss aging as though it is something that is going to happen to a select and unfortunate number of people, while they are themselves merely bystanders. In nursing, this attitude is a barrier to understanding the needs of the elderly and to providing quality care.

Exploring Nursing Attitudes

To identify and discard the myths about older people helps clear the mind and allow personal soul-searching. How do you feel about aging? Maybe you don't know. Does the way you feel about growing old have much to do with your present self-image? Is your feeling based on how you think the world will treat you when you are old?

We normally associate aging with dying, because few of us believe we will die young, and most of us wish there was some way to avoid it altogether. If we must die, we will do it when we are very old. So we don't want to get old. Furthermore, we have mental images of how many elderly people die alone and in advanced states of physical deterioration. Will this happen to us?

If a nurse is not willing to think about growing old and what it could and does mean, can she accept those people who are a reminder that aging is real? The purpose of raising these questions is to stimulate thought; answers are individual matters.

A great vocalist and advocate for creative aging, Pearl Bailey, expressed a concern felt by many older persons: "I remember when gray hair was regarded as a 'badge of honor'—when it was regarded as a sign of wisdom—where did it all go? Everyone is going to reach that point of getting older; why not respect that fact and go on with love and respect for all."

Role Models

Role models for successful aging are everywhere. Older stars of stage, screen, and politics, as well as older authors, artists, scientists and business persons, are well known to all of us. Publications for older adults, such as *Modern Maturity* and *50 Plus*, highlight older persons who are active, productive, and happy. Every community has older citizens who are still making contributions to community life. The nurse can look to the philosophies of these people to broaden her own (Fig. 1–4).

Avice Kerr, R.N., author and lecturer, was a pioneer in the field of emergency orthopedic nursing and in her 70s was self-employed as a consultant in medico-legal records in California (Fig. 1–5). Part of her philosophy of creative and productive aging is summed up in her statement on how she has accomplished so much. "It was just a matter of being where someone said, 'Why don't you . . . ?' and I could not think of any reason not to."

Exploring attitudes and feelings and formulating a philosophy about aging helps the nurse to understand the older person in sickness or in health. Concepts of health education, nursing care, and rehabilitation, as they pertain to the older individual, are more easily defined.

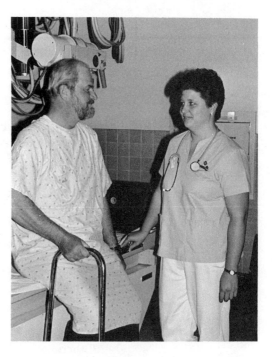

Figure 1–4. The nurse learns from older people when she tries to understand their fears and concerns.

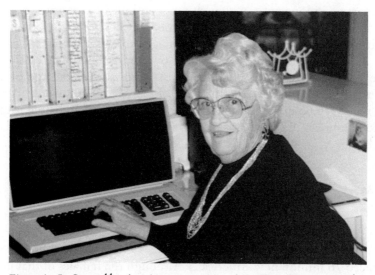

Figure 1–5. Some older Americans never retire. Avice Kerr, RN, is an author and nursing consultant in her 70s.

Aging: Toward the Future

Demographics

Decline in Death Rate

Achievements and advancements in medical, technological, and scientific fields, have made living to a ripe old age an expectation rather than a dream. At the turn of the century, life expectancy was 51 years for women and 48 years for men.

According to the U.S. National Center for Health Statistics, life expectancies for people born in 1983 are:

WOMEN:

White	78.7
Others	74.9

MEN:

White	71.7
Others	67.2

The death rate declined sharply with the conquering of infectious diseases, such as tuberculosis, smallpox, diphtheria, pneumonia and influenza, and the discoveries that made childbirth safer for both mother and baby. Better nutrition and improved living and working environments were factors in longevity. As health care continued to improve, not only did more people live longer, but the number of those living to be very old also began to increase. The 85-and-older age group is growing so fast that their number could more than double by the year 2000. According to some sources there are at least 25,000 Americans over the age of 100, whereas in 1969 there were only 3,200. Each day the number of Americans who turn 65 exceeds the death rate of the older population, causing the total number of senior citizens to swell by 1,600. One estimate claims that by the year 2000, people over age 65 will number 35 million.

Decline in Birth Rate

The steady decline in the number of babies being born in this country means a shift in the balance between the older and the younger generations. The "baby boom," which began in 1946 and lasted until 1964, produced 76 million new Americans. Although the females of that population boom have reached peak child-bearing years, the birth rate has not had a dramatic rise. The ratio of all young people to the population as a whole is dropping. Women of the baby boom generation are tending to marry later than their mothers and have fewer children, or, in many cases, none at all. In 2020, one out of every four Americans could be 65 or older.

Baby Boomer Dynamics

The first baby boomers were born right after World War II, when the United States was celebrating life, liberty, and prosperity. Getting married, settling down, and raising kids were the goals for young people, remaining so into the 1960s. Everyone knew of Dr. Benjamin Spock, pediatrician, psychiatrist, and author. His work was widely read and it served as the gospel for rearing children. Logically, pediatrics was an expanding field of practice for physicians.

Because of the 76 million children born between 1946 and 1964, emphasis in all aspects of life was placed on meeting the needs of young people. Examples of this are the television sitcoms of the '50s and '60s, which revolved exclusively around the escapades of the children and teenagers in a family. Anyone who remembers "Father Knows Best" or "Leave It To Beaver" will recall that the personalities of the parents were only revealed through meeting the needs of the children. A youth-oriented society was evolving.

As the baby boomers moved into adulthood in the early 1960s, the United States entered the conflict in Vietnam. College students and other young war protesters proclaimed that no one over 30 could be trusted. Deep rifts developed between many of these young people and their parents and other citizens.

As the baby boomers reach their 40s, it is interesting to observe the changes that are occurring in today's society. An example is the growing number of physical fitness programs for people over 40. Also, in contrast to 20 or 30 years ago, more television programs and magazines highlight older adults and their achievements and problems.

No doubt the general status of aging people will improve as the gigantic population of baby boomers begins to reach age 65. An economy geared to meeting the needs of older citizens is inevitable.

A Gerontocracy

In 2020, baby boomers will be older Americans. Americans who are now in their 50's will be the old-old people. They are a better educated and generally healthier and more active group than were their parents (Fig. 1–6). Increased life expectancy will swell their numbers.

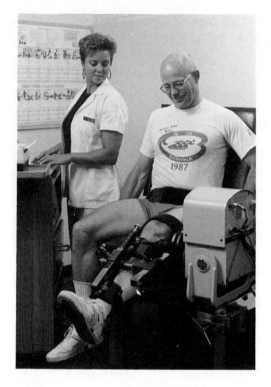

Figure 1–6. Older Americans are keeping fit and remaining active.

All signs point to a "gerontocracy," a dynamic society where older people have control. Differences in lifespan between men and women mean that this gerontocracy will be primarily comprised of women.

Trends: Making Life Better

Health Care

Increasing partnership is common among action groups of aging people and hospitals that offer streamlined services for senior citizens. One example of this cooperation is an elder care system where, for a five-dollar fee, the older person receives an identification card entitling him or her to certain privileges such as reduced prices in the hospital cafeteria. The hospital will file all claims when that person is a patient, and will accept Medicare benefits as full payment for services provided.

Within institutions, services are expanding to meet the needs of an aging population in the form of geriatric clinics, home health care agencies, outreach educational programs, senior service coordinators and even free transportation (see Fig. 1–7). Women's health centers are growing in number and focus much of their efforts on the special needs of older women, for example, cancer detection and education in the prevention and treatment of osteoporosis.

Marketing health care for older citizens is big business. From Age Wave (Emeryville, CA) has come a program called "The Role of the Hospital in an Aging Society: A Blueprint for Action," developed by Dychtwald and Zitter, two marketing consultants and experts on aging. The American Society on Aging presents seminars on marketing strategies to reach the older consumer. In general, hospital management teams are being advised that they are creating the health care system of their own future.

Housing

More attention is being given to the following options:

- Low-income housing for older people with health care services available
- Congregate or group living
- Intergenerational living — older people sharing homes with younger people, like students
- Shared housing — a small group of older persons living under one roof
- Bed, board, and care facilities

Educational Aspects

The American Association of Retired Persons (AARP), other organizations, and the federal government publish a wealth of information designed to help older people live safely and independently.

Coalitions of state aging groups plan seminars and make resources available for older adults and the general public on a variety of subjects. The Human Sciences Press, Inc., in New York, is an example of a company that makes a significant literary contribution. This press publishes the *International Journal of Technology and Aging*, insight books, periodicals, books on illness, books on ethics, books for helping children accept aging in grandparents, and books on the aging employee.

(Text continues on p. 24.)

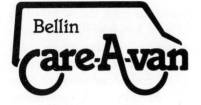

Bellin's Care-A-Van

Bellin's Care-A-Van is a free transportation service available to all Bellin Hospital patients who live within the radius indicated on the map (please see back) and are able to walk on their own or with the aid of a cane, walker, or crutches.

Whether you are traveling to or from Bellin Hospital or from your doctor's office to Bellin, let Care-A-Van be your ride.

Here's how it works:

- Call 433-7888 to schedule a time to be picked up for your appointment.
- Rides are available from 8 a.m. to 5 p.m., Monday through Friday (holidays excluded). The last van leaves the hospital at 4 p.m.
- After your appointment or stay is over, return to the Care-A-Van office (at the Clinicare entrance) to arrange for a ride home or to your doctor's office.
- One or two days advance notice is encouraged, if possible.

As you grow older, you find you're faced with many decisions when it comes to your health care. To help you with your choices Bellin Hospital has developed this directory of Services for Seniors.

In it you will find a listing of our nursing, medical, and personal services, as well as activities and educational programs for the older adult.

If you have any questions on these services or any others not listed, call our Senior Services at 433-7864.

(continued)

Figure 1–7. Many communities provide special nursing and medical services for the older adult, as well as activities and educational programs, that are similar to those described above. (Courtesy of Bellin Hospital, Green Bay, Wisconsin)

SERVICES

MEDICAL FINANCIAL ASSISTANCE

 To help you sort through your medical bills, we have designated certain staff members to work with older adults. These trained individuals from our Business Office will assist you with everything from health insurance forms to Medicare claims. If you are 65 or older, you also may be eligible for our Elder Care program. Elder Care is a cost-cutting health care plan for older adults that eliminates hospital deductibles. For more information on either of these call 433-3510.

HOME MEDICAL SUPPLIES

 All your home medical equipment needs are just a phone call away. At Bellin Hospital we offer a complete selection of home hospital equipment, such as self-help aids, ostomy supplies, walking aids, and hospital beds and accessories. Delivery and pick-up can be arranged. For more information call 433-7801.

NUTRITION SERVICES

 Our Tree Top cafeteria, located on the third floor of the hospital, offers a discount for seniors and provides a "heart healthy" menu for people with heart problems. Dietitians can also provide up-to-date information on weight management and other nutrition topics. For more information call 433-3553.

CARDIAC SERVICES

 As the only facility in northeast Wisconsin that does cardiac surgery, Bellin provides the latest diagnostic, surgical, and rehabilitation services. Our cardiac rehab program helps you return to an active and productive lifestyle. It begins while you are still in the hospital and continues on an outpatient basis once you are discharged. To learn more about our cardiac services talk to your physician.

SUPPORT GROUPS

It's hard to cope with certain situations on your own. That's why we've organized support groups in various areas that let you share your experiences with others. Stop smoking, cardiomyopathy, impotence, and respiratory support sessions are just a few that are ongoing at Bellin. All are free of charge. For more information call 433-7864.

(continued)

DIABETES EDUCATION

The purpose of our Diabetes Clinic is to teach a person to control his diabetes — not let it control him. At Bellin Hospital we teach people how to enjoy a normal, active, and healthy lifestyle. We have registered nurses and dietitians with diabetes training on hand to provide individual counseling and education for people with diabetes and their families. We also do blood sugar monitoring and foot care. To find out more call 433-3524.

HOME HEALTH CARE

Because there's no place like home, our Home Health Agency provides skilled nurses, companion sitters, home-makers, and home health aides for you or a family member who needs that special care at home. We also have a hospice program to provide support and nursing care to people who are terminally ill. Our certified and licensed Home Health Agency provides 24 hour service seven days a week. Ask your physician about home health care or call 433-3480.

THERAPY SERVICES

Our therapy services can help improve movement in arthritic joints or help you after a hip or knee replacement. We provide inpatient and outpatient services in occupational therapy, physical therapy, and at our Back School. For more information talk to your physician.

BLOOD PRESSURE SCREENING

Our Treatment Center offers free blood pressure screening daily from 3 p.m. to 8 p.m. Pre-registration is not necessary. For more information call 433-3632.

MAMMOGRAPHY

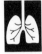

Mammography is an x-ray method used to detect lumps in the breast even before they are large enough to be felt. This safe and reliable technique is one of the most accurate methods used today. Our specially trained radiologists will analyze your mammography results and report directly to your physician. For more information contact your doctor.

PULMONARY REHABILITATION/RESTOR

RESTOR (Respiratory Education and Services Through Organized Resources) is a unique rehab program for people with chronic obstructive lung disease. You begin by attending a two-day clinic at Bellin for a diagnostic pulmonary assessment. RESTOR then works in conjunction with your physician to develop a treatment program for you to follow in your own home. Patient and family education and periodic check-ups are also included. For more information talk to your physician or call 433-3413.

(continued)

ALCOHOL AND OTHER DRUG ABUSE (AODA)

Whether alcohol or prescription drugs, addiction comes in many forms. If you or a loved one has an alcohol or drug dependency, our AODA program can provide the help that is needed. To find out more about the program contact your physician or call 433-3630.

ONE-DAY CARE/CLINICARE

Because of advancements in medical technology, some surgical procedures that use to require an overnight stay can now be performed on an outpatient basis. One-Day Care will get you in and out of the hospital in the same day, letting you recover in the comfort of your own home. Our Clinicare convenience clinic offers a low-cost, after-hours alternative to the emergency room. You will be seen by either a local physician in private practice or your personal physician for all kinds of minor injuries and illnesses. For more information on these services talk to your physician or call 433-3633.

ACTIVITIES

SENIOR U

Senior U provides ongoing educational programs that address issues such as heart disease, pre-retirement planning, and crime prevention. They also sponsor a biannual lecture that features such well-known people as Maggie Kuhn, leader of the Gray Panthers and Dr. Dean Rodeheaver, a specialist in gerontology. Recreational bus trips to plays, concerts, and shopping malls are scheduled throughout the year. Call 433-7864 for more information.

HEALTH CONNECTION

Our fitness center has many programs designed for the older adult. Senior aerobics are offered on a weekly basis, as are various dance classes. Or use our weight machines and fitness equipment to keep you limber and help combat the effects of arthritis. A certified instructor will assist you in developing a personalized program. Seniors over the age of 65 receive a discount on their membership fee to the Health Connection. For more information call 433-3638.

VOLUNTEERS

We have numerous volunteer opportunities for people of all ages at Bellin. You can work in the gift shop or information desk; dedicate your time to patient home care; help sort and deliver mail; make chaplain calls; or work directly with our patients. Whichever area you choose, you will gain self-satisfaction in donating your time and talent. If you'd like to volunteer, call 433-3469.

Advocacy

Clearly the AARP is a giant among advocates for older people. There is hardly an area of life where AARP efforts are not visible. Much of the work of this organization is done by volunteers, and the association emphasizes volunteerism as a way to help others and self. The monthly bulletin and the bimonthly publication, *Modern Maturity*, inform, entertain, and underscore the efforts of other advocates for the aging.

Agencies and political groups for the aging are growing in strength and number. One powerful group, the Gray Panthers, has a membership of over 80,000.

In church surveys of parishioners, the needs of elderly members surface in increasing numbers and with increasing frequency. As a result, many churches dedicate their resources in an effort to raise community awareness as to the needs of the elderly. They contact lawmakers with concerns, present educational conferences, and hire parish nurses who devote a major share of their time to meeting elderly parishioners' health needs.

As a community health teacher and a resource person, the nurse needs to remain updated on all of these trends and others as they develop.

Issues and Nursing Implications

Ethical

All human beings, regardless of age or health status, have the right to life. However, ethical dilemmas do arise in making life-saving decisions. Some of these issues follow:

- Do sick, dependent, and debilitated elderly people always want to live?
- Do they have the right to decide their fate?
- If they don't, who does?
- Is it ethical to use resources and technology to preserve life when the quality of that life is considered to be poor?
- Should disabled older persons be considered candidates for intensive physical rehabilitation?
- In making *any* decisions about lifesaving measures, is a judgment also being made about who is valuable and who isn't?
- How can the health care system afford to provide everyone with access to life-saving resources and technology?

These are broad issues that create ethical dilemmas when attempts are made to address them. Part of the problem is that the human race has technologically advanced itself to the point where it can assume the awesome responsibility for God-like decisions.

Ethical dilemmas may occur that will affect older people as a population. For example, some policy makers are struggling with the question of whether or not public funding for life-saving procedures, such as organ transplants, should be limited for elderly people. Unfortunately, many decisions on ethical issues will be made based on cost.

Euthanasia, often called "mercy killing," is allowing or helping a hopelessly ill person to die with relatively little suffering. Is euthanasia right or wrong? As the nation ages, this issue will be at the forefront of right-to-life, or right-to-death, decisions. The nurse is likely to be increasingly involved in situations where the term "passive euthanasia" is applied, meaning that no heroic efforts will be made to sustain life. For example, a situation may arise in which a patient with cardiac or respiratory arrest will not be resuscitated. The nurse needs to be familiar with the policies and procedures of such decision making in the institution in which she is employed (see Chap. 9).

When an older person is incapable of making choices, the family will be distressed and may feel guilty about what they consider "the right thing to do." The nurse should be as empathetic and supportive as possible. Whatever one's personal values and feelings, it is not a nurse's responsibility to pass judgment. If the nurse has strong negative feelings about the decisions made by a family or physician, she is obligated to discuss them with her immediate supervisor.

CASE STUDIES: EXAMPLES OF HOW THE NURSE COULD BECOME INVOLVED IN DECISION MAKING

Mrs. L is 83 years old and her condition has been diagnosed as inoperable bladder cancer. She has told her daughter that she does not want radiation or chemotherapy. The granddaughter is a nurse and wants to talk about this situation with the nurses who are caring for her grandmother. She says, "People are going to think we're terrible. But it's her choice isn't it? And my mother agrees with her. I don't know, what do you think?"

Mr. O is 76 years old with a "probable lung cancer," and has been examined by a specialist in respiratory disease. The pulmonary function test exhausted Mr. O to the extent that he was too tired to eat for an entire day. The only remaining diagnostic test was a lung biopsy.

Before that could take place, Mr. O was admitted to the hospital with diarrhea. Also, he had gotten out of bed to go to the bathroom at night and had fallen. The woman who has been living with him became concerned. "Otherwise," she says, "I would never have brought him in, but I was afraid he'd broken a hip." This woman has no legal right to make Mr. O's decisions, and abides by those made by the man's son and daughter. Mr. O has other chronic health problems. He is frail, weak, and has recently lost a son to heart disease. He has been depressed and does not seem to care one way or the other; he simply does what is asked of him. His remaining son and daughter want the doctor to cancel the lung biopsy. The daughter says to the nurse, "I don't think there's any way Dad could survive chemotherapy. And we don't even want to tell him about it. But you know, he saw the lung x-ray; he heard the doctor. He's no dummy. What would you do if it were your Dad?"

Health Care Financing

The broad issues here are how to control the rising costs of health care, who should pay for it, and what is the most cost-effective way to provide long-term care for older people?

Although they have been helpful in many ways, Medicare and Medicaid have not been the answer. In 1965, Medicare (Title XVIII) and Medicaid (Title XIX) became amendments to the Social Security Act. Medicare was designed to provide health-care coverage to those older people eligible for Social Security. Medicaid was meant to help persons of any age who could not pay for private health insurance, as well as those older people whose Medicare benefits had been exhausted. Medicaid is administered jointly by federal and state governments. The Veteran's Administration is one source of funding. There are deficiencies in both systems, and fraud and abuse have been widespread. Furthermore, rising health-care costs have made Medicare and Medicaid inadequate. Confusion and misconceptions generated by the procedures of these systems are enormous and too numerous to discuss here, since each person is affected in a different way. However, one popular misconception is that Medicare and Medicaid pay for all nursing home expenses. Medicare payment for nursing home expenses is limited, and families may be responsible for some nursing home costs under Medicaid.

Inadequacies in the programs account for some of these adverse developments and they raise the issue of whether or not Medicare and Medicaid should be continued. Many advocates of the elderly population believe a national health insurance program for all people is the only answer. These specific concerns and facts are related to the issues of health care financing:

1. Lack of coverage for preventive care
2. The impoverishment of one spouse while another is in a nursing home—must a couple who have been married 50 years get a divorce so that the spouse who is at home can retain his or her monthly income? Alzheimer's disease, in particular, is making old people poor.
3. The number of elderly people with chronic health problems that could deplete their financial resources
4. About 10% of all AIDS victims are over 50 years of age. Will this mean the establishment of extended care facilities with special services?

On June 8, 1988, a catastrophic health insurance bill was passed by the U.S. Senate that will provide more financial protection for the already 29 million elderly people on Medicare. The beneficiaries of services will pay the additional costs. Highlights of this bill include:

1. Full coverage of all hospital bills after an annual deductible which after 1989 may be $564
2. Full and appropriate payment of doctor bills after a $1,370 deductible
3. A 50% payment of outpatient drug costs after a $600 annual deductible, beginning in 1991

Increased home health care coverage for elderly people is still an issue of much debate.

Older persons must be educated as to the extent of medical benefits under federal, state, and private pay programs. They should have access to information about partnerships between physicians and coalitions of aging groups in which the physician accepts the Medicare assignment for a specific service rendered. The nurse's role is to know who can provide expert answers to questions about health care financing, and to stay aware of new and pending legislation (Fig. 1–8).

Care-giver Dilemmas

It's *my* home, but she's my *mother*! How am I going to tell her to clean herself up better?

Last week we had another bout with phlebitis. She would *not* let me call the doctor. If she suddenly goes with a blood clot, maybe it's for the best. I've done all I can do—but I still feel guilty.

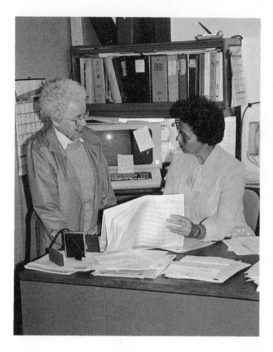

Figure 1-8. Seek expert advice about health care financing from the staff of the hospital business office.

These are the concerns of two different women, both primary care-givers to elderly mothers. They are members of the "sandwich generation," those individuals, usually women, who are sandwiched between elderly, dependent parents and adult children who have returned home to live and have needs of their own. What about the needs of the care-giver? Many of them work 40 hours a week outside the home and 20 more hours at home, just providing care. This means their own housekeeping chores and personal needs are overwhelming. The household is often crowded and conditions are stressful.

Many care-givers of elderly people have passed through middle age. It is not uncommon for a 65-year-old woman to be caring for her 90-year-old mother. An 80-year-old husband cares for an 80-year-old wife. The older care-giver may need care herself and in home health care this is very often an observation that requires attention. The issues here are who is taking care of parents and what can society do to help?

Large corporations are becoming increasingly aware that it is in their best interests to offer services to help their employees care for dependent older relatives. Staying home with a sick parent could eventually be a significant factor in absenteeism. An adult day care center might be an appealing benefit for these employees.

Elder Abuse

The physical work load, financial strain and emotional burden of caring for an elderly person can lead to mistreatment of that person. Abuse of the elderly is tragic, and those care-givers who resort to it out of exhaustion, frustration, and worry are likewise tragic, and need relief and counseling. Witnesses to elder abuse are difficult to find.

Abusers of elderly people have these characteristics:

- Usually family members; often the elderly person lives with them
- Often victims of recent stress themselves, for instance, disruptions in family life, changes in living arrangement, and loss of social support
- More likely to be suffering from financial problems, alcoholism or mental illness
- Often lacking needed services

Elder abuse takes five forms:

1. *Passive neglect*—unintentional abuse in which the care-giver does not do that which is required (such as preventing skin breakdown), due to lack of skills, knowledge or physical ability
2. *Psychological abuse*—causing mental distress by name calling, isolating, ignoring, or ridiculing the older person
3. *Financial abuse*—illegal, or unauthorized use of the person's money or property
4. *Active neglect*—deliberately abandoning an older person or denying health care
5. *Physical abuse*—inflicting pain or injury, or restraining an older person against his will

Instructing family members in caring for an elderly person in the home is an important nursing responsibility. When an older person is admitted to the hospital emergency room with a history of injury due to falls, the living conditions of that person may need to be investigated. Untreated sores or conditions may be warning signs. Older persons who appear malnourished, frightened, or depressed may be suffering from abuse. The nurse must closely observe relationships between the elderly and their family members. Care for the care-giver must become a part of long range planning for health care services for older people.

Resources to contact when elder abuse is suspected, or when families feel they *might* become abusive, are a social service agency or the police department. A crisis intervention center, often hospital-based, is another resource.

Good Intentions and Nursing Care

Older people may also suffer at the hands of their care-givers in institutional settings. Even the nurse who tries to "reason with" an elderly patient, unaware that the patient is becoming confused, may be less sensitive to feelings. Inappropriate use of restraints is abusive treatment. Doing what one *thinks* is best for the older patient does not always get the desired response if the patient is not in agreement or does not understand. Gentle persuasion turns into "you *will* do this" and this is emotionally traumatic. The most conscientious nurse may leave the elderly patient with the impression that she is "rough."

An old woman tells her niece: "I didn't like that night nurse. She made me walk to the bathroom at four o'clock in the morning. She said, 'Your doctor wants you to walk, and it's good for you.' It's *not* good for me when I'm dizzy, and I'm dizzy when I get up at night!"

The issue is that caring for elderly persons who are ill is a special kind of nursing. The nurse must have background knowledge that views the older patient as a complex human being with multiple and individual needs.

Crimes Against the Elderly

The prevalence of crime in the streets, burglary, break-ins to do bodily harm, and other forms of crime are generally more related to environment than age of the victim. Crime against the elderly is an issue for these reasons:

1. The frail elderly are especially vulnerable.
2. Many old persons live alone, especially women.
3. Older people are fearful of becoming victims of crime. They read about their peers being robbed, beaten, sexually abused, or swindled, and they are afraid it will happen to them.
4. Because they have retirement savings, older people are frequently victims of fraud, sales gimmicks, and con games, such as the following:
   - *Fraud*: A wonderful offer comes through the mail to buy some land in a warm climate, sight unseen.
   - *Sales Gimmicks*: A fear tactic is one gimmick, as when a salesman claims that a certain product or service is necessary to keep one safe from some misfortune.
   - *Con Games*: A bill comes to the widow for an expensive purchase made by the spouse, of which the widow has no recollection.

5. Elderly people who live in fear may isolate themselves, thereby decreasing the quality of their lives, and causing deterioration of their health status. For example, one might lock himself or herself in a home, and go without groceries and medical help so as not to be attacked on the street.

How does society protect older people from crime and help them to help themselves and feel safe? Local police departments have information or can get information on a multitude of subjects related to crime prevention, including how to burglarproof a home and neighborhood, how to travel safely, and how to spot consumer crimes.

In wellness promotion settings such as health fairs, the nurse can distribute information on crime prevention. The home health nurse should be alert for hints that patients and families offer that could suggest fear of some sort of crime. This is particularly true in those cases where the patient is old and the care-giver is also old.

Poverty Issues

Although many older people are financially secure, and sociologists predict this number will continue to increase, there are poverty issues in the elderly population. In 1985, over 12% of the 65+ population of the United States was below the poverty level, a slight decrease from 1983. Looking at poverty from an ethnic standpoint, there are twice as many poor, elderly Hispanics and almost three times as many poor, older blacks as there are poor, elderly whites. Poverty-stricken older females greatly outnumber poor males, and older black women have the highest incidence of poverty. Financial difficulties are a problem in low-paying jobs where retirement plans are inadequate. Obviously, the higher incidence of poverty among minorities affects the kind of health care they are able to obtain, and the poor patient may have a history of minimum or no care. The nurse must be aware of this fact when assessing needs, as this patient may need more education and greater attention to basic health care needs.

Age and Race: Discrimination and Problems

Research on aging in minority ethnic groups is difficult because of language barriers and cultural differences. The issue is to identify and reach those who need help. Some authorities state that close family structure may keep needy older Hispanics from using public resources. Families may not venture outside their own environment, preferring to solve their own problems. However, some older persons do not receive necessary care because they need better transportation to health care centers. Since the Hispanic population is growing, helping the older members to manage chronic ailments and stay as healthy as possible could become a serious problem. Attitudes and beliefs may prevent ethnic minorities from seeking medical help and health care instruction. Language barriers may contribute to misunderstanding directions and advice. Older people bring this background to the hospital with them, and the nurse must respect differences when identifying needs and giving care and instruction.

The AARP has a Minority Affairs Initiative, a minority volunteer network that seeks to help improve communication and the status of needy older people in minority groups. One way this network is approaching the problem is by reaching out to minorities through religious affiliations.

In planning for security in old age, low-income ethnic minorities are at a disadvantage because shift work and language barriers may prevent them from taking part in preretirement programs. The nurse who is employed in occupational health nursing should consider preretirement planning as wellness promotion and be aware of the difficulties ethnic minorities might have in participating.

Age discrimination in the job market has lessened in the last decade but continues to be an issue. Corporate mergers and cutbacks affect older workers, especially those in management. The nurse as a constituent can write to legislators and vote in ways that will help eliminate job discrimination against older people.

A growing concern in the future will be about the number of elderly drivers on the highway. Will more restrictions be necessary to prevent accidents that occur due to traffic violations? Or will the upcoming older generation—the baby boomers—be safer drivers, having had better training and more freeway experience? Still, there will be more drivers on the highway with decreased vision, hearing, and physical skills. The issue is open to speculation and discussion.

Substance Abuse

Of all drugs, the most widely abused is alcohol. Alcoholism is a lifelong problem for some, but many people start to drink heavily only later in life. Women are more prone to this problem than men. Alcohol offers escape from the stresses caused by crises of old age, including retirement, bereavement, poor health, and loneliness. Prolonged use of alcohol leads to depression.

The brain of the older adult is especially vulnerable to damage from alcohol, and dementia may be the result. Other problems of the aged alcoholic include the following:

- Malnutrition
- Incontinence
- Diarrhea
- Falls and injury
- Self-neglect and general physical deterioration
- Disturbance in sleep patterns with periods of agitation and irritability
- Social isolation

These signs of alcohol abuse are often mistaken for signs of aging or progression of a chronic disease. Even if they are aware of it, families may deny this problem exists, or believe that advancing age means that it is too late to do anything about it. For these reasons an older person may not get treatment.

Other age-related factors make alcohol especially hard on older people. The drug remains in the bloodstream of an older person longer than it does in a younger person and thus prolongs the deleterious effects. When alcohol is mixed with medications, they may interact with serious consequences. For instance, alcohol causes a drop in blood sugar that interferes with the body's ability to metabolize medication for diabetes.

The next most widely abused group of drugs are those that alter moods or emotions. A list of these drugs, with an example of each, follows:

- Sedatives (Equanil)
- Hypnotics (Seconal)
- Narcotics (Demerol)
- Antianxiety drugs (Valium)
- Non-narcotic analgesics (Tylenol)
- Antidepressants (Elavil)
- Antihistamines (Dristan)
- Anticholinergic drugs (Tagamet)

An awareness of the detrimental effects of substance abuse and its signs and symptoms in older persons is essential for nursing assessment. Health education for older people and their families must include information on substance abuse and the message that one *can* be, and *deserves* to be, treated at any age.

Suicide

The incidence of suicide increases after the age of 60, and the rate of suicide is highest in older men. Older people are generally successful at suicide attempts. The following are risk factors:

- Chronic painful, or disabling disease
- Loneliness and isolation
- Preoccupation with suicide, talking about it constantly
- Previous suicide attempts
- A family history of suicide
- Substance abuse
- Depression, even if the person is or has been under treatment
- Excessive feelings of guilt
- Financial problems
- Recent loss of a spouse

An important point for the nurse to remember is that an older person who talks about suicide or is severely depressed is at especially high risk.

The Frail Elderly

The frail older person is one who is probably older than 75 and requires some supportive services to cope with daily living. As advanced medical technology keeps more and more older people alive, society must be responsible for helping them achieve a high quality of life regardless of functional problems. This means that in order for older persons to remain at home, more opportunities for home help are needed. More alternatives, such as nursing homes, residences with supervised activities and prepared meals, foster homes, and adult day care centers should be made available. Support networks that offer education for self care, crisis "hot lines," and access to nursing services and supervision will be in demand. Expanded opportunities for community nursing should be an outcome of programs that seek to keep the frail elderly at home.

Issues Affecting Older Women

More older women than older men are struggling for survival in poor and unsafe living conditions, as well as acting as care-givers to adult children. Consequently, elderly women are more often the victims of neglect, abuse, and crime.

The Women's Initiative of the AARP is dedicated to making life better for older women by supporting their roles, aiding in their personal development, and recognizing their contributions to society. An older woman who wants to be involved in helping her peers might find direction by contacting this organization. The nurse will find that this organization is a resource for updated information to pass on to older women.

Summary

History and literature show evidence that there have always been mixed feelings about the value of aging. The United States has become a youth-oriented culture. In order to care for older people, the nurse must recognize that today's older population has been affected by great technological advances, wars, and economic depression. Many negative myths about aging exist and they affect the way older people are viewed and treated. Old age is not a disease that renders one sexless and senile. Most older people are well adjusted, busy, happy, and able to adapt to changing situations.

The needs of older people are increasingly being addressed in legislation and in the establishment of organizations and agencies. Demographics show that by the year 2020, this nation could become a gerontocracy in which the majority of older people are widows. Making life better for older people includes gearing health care to meet their needs and providing education. The AARP is a great advocate of older people's rights and a source of information for everyone. Health care financing is a major issue in the care of older people. The nurse will become more involved with ethical dilemmas of life or death, elder abuse, problems of care-givers, and substance abuse. Poverty, discrimination, crime, and suicide are other important issues of aging. Understanding the problems of older people will help the nurse to grow and to learn about her own future.

Activities

1. Interview an older relative in your life regarding these issues:
   a. List the major national and international events of his or her lifetime.
   b. Question that person about memories of those events, including roles, feelings, and values — the relative's own and those of people he or she knows. Try to reconstruct, for example, what life was like in a specific family and neighborhood during World War II.
   c. Obtain a history of childhood diseases.
   d. Ask about elderly people your relative remembers. Who were they and what were their backgrounds?
   e. List technological developments in his lifetime as he or she remembers them.
2. Find a current newspaper or magazine article that discusses a trend or issue related to aged persons and their needs. Bring the article to class for discussion.

3. Select one of the following activities and report on it to the class:
   a. Contact your local police department and ask for literature on how senior citizens can protect themselves against crime.
   b. Interview a hospital administrator on long-range planning for special services for older people.
   c. Interview the manager of an apartment building designed for senior citizens to find out the average age of tenants, how many are older women living alone, availability of apartments, and plans for the future.
   d. Interview an intensive care nurse about ethical issues involving elderly patients and any experiences and feelings the nurse is willing to share related to the subject.
   e. Discuss an ethical issue that could arise concerning an older person in your own family.
4. Complete the following:
   a. When I think about old people, I think about _____.
   b. I hope to live to be _____ years old.
   c. Two good things about old age are _____

   _____

   _____.
   d. Two bad things about old age are _____

   _____

   _____.
   e. When I am 80 I want to _____.
   f. The world needs old people to _____.
   g. I will be different than my grandparents because _____

   _____

   _____.
   h. Finding a way to stop aging would be (good or bad) because

   _____.
   i. Old people should be taken care of by _____.
   j. When I am 80 the world will be _____.
   k. Older men and older women are different because _____

   _____

   _____.
   l. Older men and older women are alike because _____

   _____

   _____.
5. "What Will I Look Like?" Is there a connection between how we think our appearance will change and how we feel about growing older? Possibly. Try this exercise:

Stand in front of a mirror and take some time to think about an older person in your family whom you resemble. Now look closely at your reflection and imagine, in detail, how your face, hair, body structure, and posture will become like theirs. Where will you be grayest? Where will the wrinkles in your face be? Will you be fatter, thinner, stooped? Picture how that person's hands look, if you can, and look at your hands, and see them as they will look when you get older. Construct as much of that family member's image on your own image as you can. How do you feel about what you have just done? Why?

6. Describe an older person whom you consider a role model. Why do you admire this person?

Bibliography

Barash D: Aging. An Exploration. Seattle, University of Washington Press, 1983
Bock K, Schilder E: Physical restraints. Can Nurse 84:34–37, 1988
Burnside I: Nursing and the Aged. A Self-Care Approach, 3rd ed. New York, McGraw-Hill, 1988
Butler R: Geriatrics in action. Getting older and getting better. Healthcare Executive, March/April:24–27, 1987
Butler R: The longevity revolution. Mt Sinai J Med 54:5–8, 1987
Carlson R: Adult rehabilitation attitudes and implications. J Gerontol Nurs 14:25–30, 1988
Cody M: Withholding treatment: is it ethical? J Gerontol Nurs 12:24–26, 1986
Dolan M: Meet the "chronologically gifted." Nursing 17:56–57, 1987
Dychtwald K, Zitter M: The elderly as healthcare consumers. Healthcare Executive Vol. 2, 1987
Dychtwald K: The truth about elders. Health Care Forum Vol. 30, 1987
Dychtwald K: Wellness and Health Promotion for the Elderly. Rockville, MD, Aspen, 1986
Ebersole P, Hess P: Toward Healthy Aging. Human Needs and Nursing Response, 2nd ed. St. Louis, CV Mosby, 1985
Lasker M: Aging alcoholics need nursing help. J Gerontol Nurs 12:21–24, 1986
National Association for Home Care: Caring, Vol. 6, No. 9. Washington, DC, 1987
Penn C: Promoting independence. J Gerontol Nurs 14:14–19, 1988
Pifer A, Bronte L (ed): Our Aging Society. Paradox and Promise. New York, WW Norton and Co, 1986
Rice L: Do we discriminate against the elderly? Nursing 18:44–45, 1988
Roberts A: Systems of life, No. 157: Senior systems. 22, Nurs Times, 84:49–52, 1988
Rose J: When the care plan says restrain. Geriatr Nurs 8:20–21, 1987
Scott R: Dilemmas in practice: When it isn't life or death . . . when the aging parents can no longer live independently (case study). Am J Nurs 85:19–20, 1985
Slack P: Sweet Adeline. Nurs Times 84:25–29, 1988
Strumpf N: A new age for elderly care. Nurs & Health Care 8:444–448, 1987
Thobaben M: Abuse: The shameful secret of elder care. RN 51:85–86, 1988

Tierney J et al: And don't send her back! Agitated nursing home residents are dumped in the E.R. Am J Nurs 86:1011–1014, 1986

US Dept. of Commerce, Bureau of the Census: 1987 Statistical Abstract of the United States, 107th ed. Selected Life Table Values, 1959–1983, p. 70. Washington, DC, 1987

World Almanac and Book of Facts. New York, A Scripps Howard Co, 1987

Youngberg B: When the patient has been battered. Nursing 15:32c–32h, 1985

2

Nursing the Aging Person: Development and Process

Learning Objectives

When you complete this chapter, you should be able to:

1. *Write three general comments about the history of nursing the aged.*
2. *Differentiate between "geriatrics" and "gerontology."*
3. *Identify the steps in the nursing process, along with a comment for each about special considerations for an elderly patient.*
4. *Give specific reasons why an admission interview must be detailed.*
5. *Define "nursing diagnoses."*
6. *Write a functional assessment of an elderly person in your life.*
7. *Describe the general levels of care in nursing homes.*
8. *Discuss nursing roles in the care of aging people.*

The history of nursing and a concern for the welfare of older people are inseparable. Nursing itself is as old as the human feelings of sympathy and love, and as new as the concepts and discoveries that constantly influence its development.

Although nursing homes have always presented opportunities for the nurse who wishes to work with older people, the aging of society is increasing those opportunities and is affecting and expanding the roles of the nurse in other areas.

Care of the Aged: A Historical Overview

Early History

In those primitive and ancient cultures where aged members were valued, women must have nurtured and cared for the aging in the same way they cared for the young. According to nursing history textbooks, the early Christian Church in Europe assumed responsibility for social services, which included offering assistance to the aged. Nursing was a primary function of nuns and other groups of religious women, and a task of monks. The Crusades and the Holy Wars of the Middle Ages (500–1500 A.D.) created a multitude of widows, and it was common for women to form lay communities to care for the less fortunate, including the elderly, who were often without other resources.

In the 16th century, the Protestant Reformation also took place. Many charitable hospitals under the direction of Catholic religious orders had to cease operation, and the poor, the aged, the sick, and the orphaned were deprived of a primary source of care. Conditions in public hospitals did not improve until the late 18th and early 19th centuries.

The Influence of Florence Nightingale

Florence Nightingale, the founder of professional nursing, was a humanitarian with an interest in people of all ages. Commitment to the comfort and care of the sick and a concern for their environment and overall quality of life was her definition of nursing. Her nurses went out into the communities of Great Britain and into the almshouses, or poorhouses. Here the poor, chronically ill, mentally afflicted, and dependent old were thrown together and cared for by inmates committed to the same building for minor criminal offenses. Many Nightingale nurses were leaders in improving conditions at those institutions and organizing other humanitarian groups who helped establish training programs for district nurses. The dependent aged, although few in number, were among the needy who benefited from this nursing service.

The Origin of Geriatric Care

An English physician and author, Trevor H. Howell, tells an interesting story in his book, *Our Advancing Years*. He writes about an incident in an almshouse in Vienna in the late 1880s. A group of medical students are visiting their instructor, who has just finished demonstrating certain aspects of disease in some of the patients:

> Just as he was going, however, an old woman hobbled up to him and complained of her aches and pains. "Oh, you are just suffering from old age," he said. One of the students asked what could be done for such a case. "Nothing," was the pessimistic reply. This answer made a deep impression on Ignatz Nascher, one of the young men who were present. The woman was suffering from old age and nothing could be done to relieve her! Was old age, then, a disease from which those who reached advanced life were doomed to suffer? He pondered long over the incident. At length, he decided that there could be no justification for such an attitude of hopelessness. When this young man became a qualified doctor of medicine, he devoted himself to the study of disease in elderly patients.

From the Greek word *gēras*, meaning "old age," Dr. Nascher coined the word "geriatrics." Thirty years later, in 1914, he published a book called *Geriatrics: The Diseases of Old Age and Their Treatment*.

Despite the increasing population of elderly people, geriatrics as a specialty has grown slowly (Fig. 2–1). In 1986, the number of qualified physician-geriatricians in this country was about 100. Geriatric nursing,

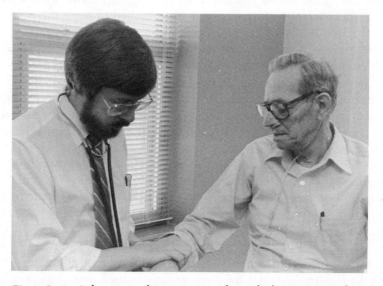

Figure 2–1. A doctor trained in geriatrics understands the importance of time and patience.

in any setting, is still regarded by many nurses as depressing and uninteresting.

Definitions of Gerontology

"Gerontology" is the study of the aged at a scientific, psychological, social, or philosophical level. The development of this field is closely linked to political activity, because of federal funding and legislation for aging issues.

Scientific research into the process of aging is concerned with learning how and why the human organism undergoes change with age. Numerous theories of aging have been advanced, some of which will be discussed in Chapter 3.

In the field of psychology, gerontology is comparatively new. It has been difficult for psychologists to study healthy older adults and come to conclusions about them because each person ages in a different way.

Social gerontology is concerned with the roles of the elderly in society. Research and debate center around potential useful roles and decision-making functions of older people. Philosophical studies of aging have to do with understanding the meaning of life on a personal level.

Past Trends in Nursing

In 1935, when Social Security was introduced, the emphasis in nursing was on caring for the ill elderly. This was logical because nurses came from hospital schools of nursing and were trained to meet the needs of hospitals.

The concept of caring for the elderly in boarding houses or convalescent homes can be traced back to early American history. Licensed facilities began to appear in the 1930s and 1940s. Due to attitudes about aging, nursing homes were looked upon, in general, as substandard institutions in which to practice nursing. Nonprofessional care-givers were often poorly prepared for the task of caring for ill and dependent residents. Standards of care left much to be desired.

By 1950, references to geriatrics were included in some basic nursing textbooks, but geriatric nursing was not given much attention. Aging was not generally presented as a normal process with potential problems and implications for preventive nursing. In one hospital school of nursing, a suggested approach to the care of the ill elderly was to "treat them as if they are your own grandparents." Elderly people were being treated and cared for, no matter how kindly, as having outlived their usefulness. Few nurses had an interest in a field where hopelessness was the prevailing attitude and challenge was absent.

Nursing literature of the 1960s discussed the increasing population of older persons. Aging was equated with an increased incidence of degenerative joint disease and chronic illness. The need for a wellness component in health care planning was lacking. Textbooks discussed the growing number of older people as a strain on health care resources. Projections for the future suggested the need for more home health care agencies and long-term care facilities.

Development of Gerontological Nursing Practice

In 1966, the American Nurses' Association (ANA) established a Division of Geriatric Nursing. Its goals would be to upgrade and advance the practice of geriatric nursing, and to develop nurses in this specialty. Institutional care would be improved to meet new standards. Nursing home nurses, especially, welcomed this development. In 1970, medical-surgical nursing textbooks were presenting care plans for nursing older patients that took into account the specific problems of aging.

In 1976, the Division of Geriatric Nursing became the Division of Gerontological Nursing, because promoting wellness in the elderly had become a nursing goal. Standards of Gerontological Nursing Practice were developed by this new division and serve as guidelines for the nursing care of older adults. Standards of care are a model for the nurse to follow. They identify *what* must be done to plan and provide nursing care, determine if that care is effective, and change and update plans.

How these things are accomplished is decided by using the nursing process (see pp. 45–50). Standards of nursing are also used as a method of comparison and evaluation by those who make judgments on quality of care.

Nursing Research in Gerontology

In 1985, the Cabinet on Nursing Research of the ANA listed the following questions as research areas in health care of the elderly*:

1. How do the health needs (physical, psychological, social, and spiritual) of the elderly differ from those of other age groups?
2. How have the changing patterns of families influenced the health and health care of the elderly?
3. What productive roles can the elderly fulfill in society?
4. How can family members be assisted in coping with the health needs of their elderly members?

*American Nurses' Association, Cabinet on Nursing Research. Directions for Nursing Research: Toward the Twenty-first century, 1985, with permission.

5. What settings (currently existing or proposed) can provide effective health care for the elderly?
6. What nursing interventions and implementation processes will effectively meet the health needs of the elderly?
7. What is the role of the elderly in promoting their own health and preventing illnesses? How can this role of health promotion and illness prevention be expanded?
8. How have life-styles (such as poverty or positive and negative health habits) and environment (such as technological advances) affected the health of the elderly?

Human Needs of the Aging Person

One goal of nursing care is to help a person to meet certain basic needs. The nurse does this by assisting that person to help himself, by acting on his behalf, and by giving hands-on care. Basic needs, as identified by the psychologist, Maslow, have been placed in a hierarchy (see Fig. 2–2).

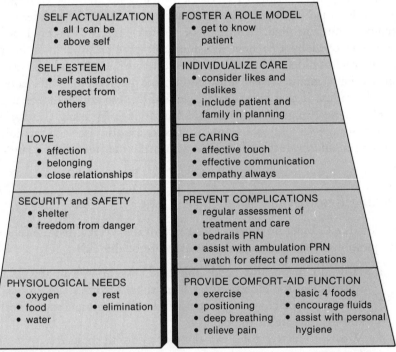

Figure 2–2. Maslow's hierarchy of needs and their implications for the nursing care of older persons.

Maslow stated that one must satisfy simple physiological needs before moving on to needs for emotional and creative fulfillment.

Nursing actions, according to this hierarchy, must be directed toward doing *first things first*. When physiological needs are met, the elderly patient is comfortable and more cooperative. For example, keeping an elderly incontinent patient dry promotes rest. A well-rested patient is more likely to engage in activities that prevent complications of immobility, such as thrombophlebitis, pneumonia, urinary stasis, and constipation. Preventing complications is part of meeting the need for safety.

The nurse communicates caring by her actions as well as words, which will be more meaningful to the elderly patient who, for example, is resting in a dry bed after walking in the hallway and having a glass of fruit juice. The nurse contributes, step by step, to meeting the elderly person's need for love.

The Nursing Process: Definition and Purpose

The nursing process is the orderly collection of information about a patient and the effective use of this information to plan, carry out, and evaluate nursing care. There are five steps in the nursing process and they are continually repeated in a cycle of nursing actions, as the nurse solves problems and meets needs. Although this is a nursing process, it involves other health care-givers, the patient, and the patient's family or other responsible persons.

In caring for elderly patients, the input of significant others is especially important. For example, Mrs. H is 80 years old and has had a total hip replacement. Two days after surgery, she begins having nausea and vomiting. Stopping her pain medications and antibiotics does not solve the problem. She has no history of stomach or bowel disorders. When the nurse approaches the daughter in the hallway to ask if she has any idea as to what may be happening, the daughter tells her, "My mother always gets nauseated when she's nervous, and she's nervous about going to therapy."

Steps in the Nursing Process

Step I. Patient Assessment (Fig. 2–3)

Collecting information or data about the patient and identifying problems requires the following steps:

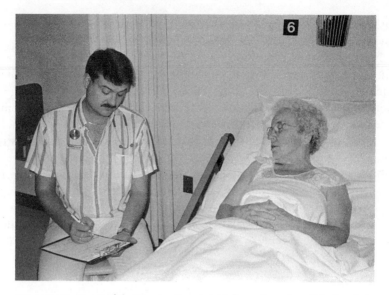

Figure 2–3. Step I of the Nursing Process includes an interview of the hospitalized patient.

- Completing an admission interview
- Conducting physical examination
- Reading reports and the notes of others
- Referring to written resources as necessary
- Using one's own nursing knowledge to analyze information
- Stating the patient's problems or potential problems as nursing diagnoses

In-depth assessment will provide clues to recent stress the older patient may have experienced and has been reluctant to mention. For example, Mr. J is 72 years old and is admitted to the hospital by rescue squad with headaches and dizziness after he "blacked out for a while." By asking questions about his family, and where they live, the nurse learns that his 17-year-old grandson was killed in a recent car accident. This will be a consideration in assessing his symptoms, his moods, and his interactions.

Misunderstandings about medications, past treatments, and medical advice often come to light in the course of an interview. In this way, the nurse learns about the elderly patient's health education needs.

Step II. Nursing Diagnoses

The nurse analyzes information and develops *nursing diagnoses*. These diagnoses describe the problems that interfere with meeting the patient's basic needs, along with possible contributing factors. Nursing diagnoses are recorded on the care plan and are the basis for establishing goals and planning care. A nursing diagnosis gives all of the team members a point of reference to explain *why* a specific plan is in place, and it assists them in making observations.

For example, an older patient often has *impaired physical mobility*, and will either be unable to ambulate or will require assistance. When the nurse makes a decision about the reason for this limitation, and states this in a nursing diagnosis, nursing care can be more patient-directed.

Let us consider two different patients. One had heart disease and this diagnosis:

"Impaired physical mobility related to pain, fatigue, edema, and medication."

The other patient has a neurological problem with this nursing diagnosis:

"Impaired physical mobility related to weakness, vertigo, and poor coordination."

Although both patients will have a nursing order to be ambulated with assistance, the assistance will be different. The neurological patient will have a cane. The cardiac patient needs a nurse at his side and holding his arm. Other orders for care and observations will also vary in accordance with the factors that cause the limitations of these patients. For instance, after ambulating, the patient with heart disease may need to have his lower extremities elevated to decrease edema.

A list of accepted nursing diagnoses is constantly being updated by the North American Nursing Diagnosis Association (see pp. 48–50). This system of identifying problems that call for specific nursing actions make patient care more consistent and complete.

Step III. Planning Care

Before the nurse can plan care, goals should be established. Goals are patient behaviors or expectations that indicate the problem has been solved or prevented. Whenever possible, the patient should help set these goals. Goals must be specific and realistic, and they must relate to the nursing diagnoses:

- *Short-term goals* — to be met in the hospital, in a matter of hours or days. Example: The patient will independently drink six glasses of water every day.
- *Long-term goals* — what the patient hopes will eventually happen. Example: The patient will weigh 150 pounds by (date). (20 pounds weight loss in 4 months)

(Text continues on p. 50.)

APPROVED NURSING DIAGNOSES, NORTH AMERICAN NURSING DIAGNOSIS ASSOCIATION, 1988

Activity intolerance
Activity intolerance, potential
Adjustment, impaired
Airway clearance, ineffective
Anxiety
Aspiration, potential for
Body image disturbance
Body temperature, altered, potential
Bowel incontinence
Breastfeeding, ineffective
Breathing pattern, ineffective
Cardiac output, altered: Decreased (specify)
Communication, impaired: Verbal
Constipation
Constipation, colonic
Constipation, perceived
Coping, family: Potential for growth
Coping, ineffective, family: Compromised
Coping, ineffective, family: Disabling
Coping, ineffective, individual
    Defensive coping
    Ineffective denial
Decisional conflict (specify)
Diarrhea
Disuse syndrome, potential for
Diversional activity, deficit
Dysreflexia
Family process, altered
Fatigue
Fear
Fluid volume excess
Fluid volume deficit
Fluid volume deficit, potential
Gas exchange, impaired
Grieving, anticipatory
Grieving, dysfunctional
Growth and development, altered
Health maintenance, altered
Health-seeking behaviors (specify)
Home maintenance, impaired
Hopelessness

**APPROVED NURSING DIAGNOSES, NORTH AMERICAN
NURSING DIAGNOSIS ASSOCIATION, 1988 (*continued*)**

Hyperthermia
Hypothermia
Incontinence, functional
Incontinence, reflex
Incontinence, stress
Incontinence, total
Incontinence, urge
Infection, potential for
Injury, potential for (specify): suffocation, poisoning, trauma
Knowledge deficit (specify)
Mobility, impaired physical
Noncompliance (specify)
Nutrition, altered: Less than body requirements
Nutrition, altered: More than body requirements
Nutrition, altered: Potential for more than body requirements
Oral mucous membrane, altered
Pain
Pain, chronic
Parental role conflict
Parenting, altered
Parenting, altered: Potential
Personal identity disturbance
Post trauma response
Powerlessness
Rape trauma syndrome
Rape trauma syndrome: Compound reaction
Rape trauma syndrome: Silent reaction
Role performance, altered
Self-care deficit: Bathing/hygiene
Self-care deficit: Dressing/grooming
Self-care deficit: Feeding
Self-care deficit: Toileting
Self-esteem disturbance
    Chronic low self-esteem
    Situational low self-esteem
Sensory/perceptual alteration: Visual, auditory, kinesthetic, gustatory, tactile, olfactory
Sexual dysfunction
Sexuality patterns, altered
Skin integrity, impaired: Actual

(continued)

**APPROVED NURSING DIAGNOSES, NORTH AMERICAN
NURSING DIAGNOSIS ASSOCIATION, 1988 (*continued*)**

Skin integrity, impaired: Potential
Sleep pattern disturbance
Social interaction, impaired
Social isolation
Spiritual distress (distress of the human spirit)
Swallowing, impaired
Thermoregulation, ineffective
Thought processes, altered
Tissue integrity, impaired
Tissue perfusion, altered: (specify) cerebral, cardiopulmonary, renal,
    gastrointestinal, peripheral
Unilateral neglect
Urinary elimination, altered patterns
Urinary retention
Violence, potential for: Self-directed or directed at others

The nurse decides what kind of nursing actions *could* be taken and then selects those she judges to be the most workable. These are written as nursing orders on the care plan. This is an example of a nursing order: Encourage the patient to drink a glass of water at 8 A.M. – 10 – 12 – 2 – 4 – 6 P.M.

Step IV. Implementations

The nurse puts the care plan into action. Besides giving care, the nurse must observe how the patient is responding. Nursing actions and patient responses are accurately and clearly charted.

Step V. Evaluating Care

The nurse reviews the goals and checks patient progress as documented in the chart and by further patient assessment. The plan is updated with new nursing orders as necessary.

The Admission Interview

When an older person is admitted to the hospital, the nurse must remember these points:

- More time is needed to interview someone with a health history that spans well over 50 years.

- Age-related changes slow responses.
- Older people do not always regard the events in their health history as important enough to mention. Either the event was "too long ago" to make a difference, or they have adapted to any problems that resulted.

For this reason, information from an interview should be validated with a significant other. Beginning with the chief complaint, a guide to asking questions on admission follows.

Interviewing An Older Patient

Reasons for Admission or Chief Complaints

Ask the patient to describe in his own words, whenever possible, the reason he came to the hospital:

- What is the problem or problems?
- When did it happen or begin?
- With every symptom or complaint, ask: Where is it? How severe is it? How often does it happen and at what times? How long does it last? What makes it better or worse?

Health History

- What is your general health now?
- Do you have any chronic problems, such as diabetes, high blood pressure, or heart disease?
- Obtain weight, height, and vital signs — has there been any weight loss?
- Do you wear glasses, a hearing aid, or dentures? Describe hearing loss and any vision loss.
- Do you use a cane, crutches, or walker?
- Do you have any pain, unusual sensations, or lack of sensation?
- Do you have any cough, shortness of breath, other trouble breathing, or with sputum?
- Are there any headaches, dizziness, weakness, fainting spells, or excessive sweating?
- Is there any swelling?
- Are there any discharges or drainage from anywhere?
- Does your heart ever race, pound, or seem to skip a beat?
- What childhood diseases did you have? (for example, measles)

- Were you immunized, that is, given shots or vaccinated, for any diseases? How about shots for lockjaw or tetanus?
- As an adult, what illnesses have you had that came and went, such as pneumonia or blood clots?
- Were you ever treated for any mental problems, like depression?
- What operations have you had?
- Did you ever injure yourself and then receive treatment? Do you ever fall?
- Were you ever in the hospital for any other reason?
- Tell me all the medications you take for any reason; prescription, over-the-counter, or any home remedies. (Collect all medications. If the patient has left any prescription drugs at home, make arrangements to have them brought in.)
- Has the doctor ever told you that you had any allergies to medicine, such as penicillin? Do you have any other allergies?
- Do you have any problems eating, such as trouble swallowing, or nausea or vomiting after eating?

General Health Habits

- Are you on a special diet? What foods do you normally eat?
- Do you drink coffee or tea?
- How many glasses of water do you drink in one day?
- How many hours do you usually sleep at night? Do you take naps? Do you have any trouble sleeping? What kind of trouble?
- Do you bathe daily? Do you prefer shower or tub?
- What are your bowel habits? Do you use laxatives, suppositories, or enemas? Do you ever have diarrhea?
- Tell me about your bladder habits: Do you urinate often during the day? In small amounts or fairly large amounts? Do you have any problems urinating? Do you get up at night to go to the bathroom?
- Do you exercise? How and how often?
- Do you drink any alcoholic beverages? If so, what kind and how often?
- Do you smoke? If so, what and how often?
- Tell me about your memory.

Family History

Ask about the age and health of all living relatives, and the age and cause of death of the others. It is important to observe carefully the older patient who is relating the causes of death of parents or siblings. Often this is a source of great fears, and it helps explain a patient's behaviors. For example, if a 69-year-old woman had one sister and one brother who died of cancer, she may be fearful that her present symptoms indicate cancer.

Psychosocial History (Assessment of Level of Functioning)

- Where and with whom do you live?
- Do you have stairs to climb?
- What do you do on an average day?
- Do you have help with anything? Describe.
- Are you satisfied with the way you can do things, or do you feel you could use more help?
- Do you get out regularly? What kinds of things do you do?
- Do you attend a certain church?

Functional assessment tells the nurse how the older person was getting along in their environment. It is a history of capabilities, that is, what can or could they do *before* they entered the hospital. This is the baseline for the functional assessment that will precede discharge. At that time, what must be decided is whether the elderly patient can remain independent or has become partially or totally dependent. Other significant questions may be these: What kind of work did you do in the past? Have you always lived in this area? Is your family close by?

Basic Methods of Physical Examination

Some of the information on an admission data base is obtained by physical examination. There are four basic methods the nurse can use. They are:

1. *Inspection* — Looking is a major part of assessment. The patient must be carefully looked at, in head-to-toe inspection. Observing the patient's reactions during examination and interview is also part of inspection.
2. *Palpation* — To palpate is to examine by feeling or touching.
3. *Auscultation* — To auscultate is to listen with a stethoscope.
4. *Percussion* — In this method of examination, the nurse uses the fingertips to tap lightly and firmly.

Other Assessment Considerations

Nursing assessment of the older patient may be more or less extensive in some areas than others when that patient is being admitted to a nursing home. For example, a psychosocial interview will not be as detailed for the patient who is not expected to leave a nursing home. However, the functional ability of that patient, now a "resident," will be very carefully assessed. Daily routines will be important to the care plan. Knowing mental status and memory will aid the nurse in communicating with the older person. See Figures 2–4 and 2–5 on the following pages for sample admission assessment forms. Note the differences between the hospital form and the form from the nursing center.

Interviewing and examining the patient is an ongoing process that is the responsibility of all team members. Hands-on care presents an excellent opportunity for the nurse to assess the patient in response to his complaints and to observe the results of nursing actions.

CASE STUDY

Mr. O is 80 years old. He has been in the hospital for two days undergoing extensive tests to diagnose the cause of a possible bowel obstruction. He has a continuous IV and, therefore, needs assistance with bathing. His abdomen is auscultated once each shift and, so far, his bowel sounds have been absent or faint. When the L.P.N. has helped him with his bath, he complains of a "new" cramp. The L.P.N. should auscultate his abdomen, palpate for tenderness, observe for distention, and then report his complaint along with her findings to the R.N.

Evaluation of Care

Patient care, and the effectiveness of the plan, is evaluated at these times:

- At least once during each shift, in order to report and chart
- Whenever a change occurs in the patient
- When it is time to compare the patient's response to a short-term goal

Evaluation results in further assessment and new nursing diagnoses and orders. The input of all team members is imperative in evaluating care. Team conferences are helpful.

(Text continues on p. 60.)

NURSING HISTORY & ASSESSMENT

Informant(s): _____

Date/Time Assessment Completed: _____

Signature of R.N. Completing: _____

Other nurses involved in gathering data: _____

Nursing Diagnoses/Problems Identified:
_____
_____
_____
_____

Admitting Medical Diagnoses (see PPOC):

Other Illnesses or Conditions (past hospitalizations, surgeries, injuries, etc.):	Allergies (food, medicine, tape, etc.)	Type of reaction:
Reason for Nursing Home Admission:		

Current Medication Taken (Prescribed & OTC)	Amount/Frequency Taken	Time Last Taken	Resident's Understanding of Purpose

Recent Laboratory Data:

Mental Status & Behaviors:

Level of Consciousness:	Level of Orientation:	Memory:
Alert: _____	Person: _____	Immediate: _____
Semicomatose: _____	Place: _____	Recent Past: _____
Comatose: _____	Time: _____	Distant Past: _____

Behaviors: (cooperative, agitated, combative, self-injurious, wandering, etc.)
_____
_____
_____

Special Precautions (describe): _____

	Resident Care Ability				RESTRAINTS: Type Ordered:
	Self	Assist.	Total	Comment	
Feeding	____	____	____	____	When to be used:
Toileting	____	____	____	____	
Grooming	____	____	____	____	
Bathing	____	____	____	____	
Mobility	____	____	____	____	Physician:
	____	____	____	____	

Usual Routines: (Sleep, meal & activity patterns)	Admission Date: LOC:
Day:	DOB: Marital Status:
PM:	ID # Room #:
NOC:	Resident:

(Continued)

Figure 2–4. An example of a nursing home history and assessment form.

	INFORMATION GATHERED FROM RESIDENT/INFORMANT:	NURSING EXAMINATION/INSPECTION
Vision/Hearing/Speech	Limitations or impairment related to: Vision ☐ YES ☐ NO Hearing ☐ YES ☐ NO Speech ☐ YES ☐ NO Describe limitation:	Appearance of eyes and ears: describe speech, language spoken Glasses _____ Contact Lenses_____ Artificial eye _____ Hearing Aid _____ Communication aid or device _____
Skin	Reported lesions, rashes, sensitivities, surgical wounds, etc.:	Inspection for condition & open areas. Include hair and nails: Decubitus location/size in cm: Presence/character of drainage:
Nutrition/Hydration	Reports of ability to chew and swallow, recent change in weight, appetite, adaptive equipment, etc.:	Skin turgor, appearance of mouth, condition of teeth, gastrostomy, N/G, IV: Diet Order: _____ Dentures: Height: Weight:
Elimination	Elimination habits, constipation, menstrual discomfort, etc.: Menstruation: Last MP: Last BM: Last Procto:	Bowel sounds, appearance of stool, urine, catheter, ostomy, incontinent, etc.:
Circulation	Reports of pain, numbness, tingling in chest or limbs, swelling, etc.:	Color, temp., edema, absence of hair, heart rate & rhythm, murmurs, etc.: _____ Temp: ____ ☐ Oral ☐ Rectal ☐ Ax B/P: __ Pulses: _____ Apical _____ Radial _____ Pacer: Set Rate:
Movement	Reports difficulty with ambulation, mobility, transfers, etc.:	ROM, gait, transfers, contractures, amputation, etc.: Cane _____ W/C _____ Walker _____ Prosthesis _____ Braces _____ _____
Pain/Discomfort	Report of pain, location, severity, causative factors, duration & how relieved:	Observed signs of pain—guarding, grimacing, etc.
Breathing	Report of dyspnea, cough, wheezing, etc.: Smoking history:	Breath sounds, Oxygen use, trach, etc.: Resp. rate: _____

SPECIAL COMMENTS/OBSERVATIONS:

NURSING ADMISSION INTERVIEW

Date	Time	Emergency Phone Numbers:	
Mode of Admission		Name	Phone
BP: R ___ ☐ Lying ☐ Standing L ___ ☐ Sitting	Pulse ___ ☐ Ap. ☐ Radial ☐ Reg. ☐ Irreg.	Name	Phone
		Family MD	
Respirations	Temp. ☐ Po ☐ R ☐ Ax	I.D. Band	Oriented to
Height	Weight: Stated	Applied	Room/Policies
	Scale	Medicare Notice Given	
Labs UA CXR		Valuables & Disposition	
Information Obtained from:			

HEALTH PERCEPTION — HEALTH MANAGEMENT   Completed By: _____

Reason for Admission (Pts. Words)

History of Present Condition

Medical History/Exposure to Communicable Diseases

Past Surgeries

Family History of Disease

MEDICATIONS   Disposition: _____

Medication & Dosage Purpose	Times — Circle Last Dose	Medication & Dosage Purpose	Times — Circle Last Dose

ALLERGIES AND REACTIONS

Drug	Past Blood Reaction
	Allergy Name Band Applied
Food	Chart & Kardex Labeled
Other	Entered in Computer allergies or no known allergies

PATIENT PROFILE   Indicate if * items were brought into the hospital

Last Food/Drink	Smoking Habits	* Glasses/Contact Lenses
Special Diet	Alcohol Usage	* Assist Devices
HX Anesthesia Problems?	Street Drug Usage	* Prosthesis
Family/Friend with Pt?	* Dentures	* Hearing Aid

Short Stay Patients Stop Here   Signature _____

(Continued)

Figure 2–5. Above is an example of a hospital form to be completed during a nursing admission interview. (Courtesy of Bellin Hospital, Green Bay, Wisconsin)

57

COGNITIVE PERCEPTUAL PATTERN

LOC/Orientation	Seizures
Pupils	Dizziness
	Fainting
Speech	Visual Impairment
Taste/Smell	Hearing Impairment
Memory	Perception of Pain (0–5 Scale)
Headaches	
Hallucinations	Do you have any special learning needs?
Additional Data:	

ACTIVITY EXERCISE PATTERN   Rt.   Lt.

Exercise Pattern	Motion & Strength Extremities
Ability to Ambulate & do ADL's	Radial Pulses
Occupation & Interests	Pedal Pulses
	Numbness/Tingling Extremities
Breath Sounds	Joint Pain
Edema	Fractures/Loss of Body Part
Cough	
Sputum	Allen's Test
Orthopnea	Skin Color
Dyspnea	Skin Temp.
Heart Sounds	
Diaphoresis	
Chest Pain & Associated SX	
Additional Data:	

SLEEP   REST   PATTERN

Sleep Pattern	Dreams/Nightmares
Nighttime Rituals	
Additional Data:	

NUTRITIONAL   METABOLIC   PATTERN

Diet/Meal Pattern	Nausea/Vomiting
	Swallowing Ability
Appetite	Oral Mucosa/Gums/Teeth
Weight Loss or Gain	
Abdomen	Skin (Turgor, Dryness, Lesions, Ecchymosis, Birthmarks)
Bowel Sounds	
Excessive Hunger/Thirst	
Additional Data:	

(Continued)

58

ELIMINATION PATTERN

Bowel Pattern	Last BM	Urine Color & Frequency
Diarrhea		Hematuria
Constipation		Burning/Hesitancy
Laxative Use		Nocturia
Additional Data:		

SEXUALITY   REPRODUCTIVE PATTERN

Menstrual Pattern/LMP	Penile Discharge
Number of Children	Lesions
Vaginal Discharge	Testicular Pain
Last Pelvic/Pap Smear	Testicular Swelling
Self Breast Exam	Testicular Self Exam
Additional Data:	

SELF PERCEPTION   ROLE RELATIONSHIPS   COPING

Pts. Description of Self	Family/Support Systems
Emotional State	Financial Concerns
Recent Stressors in Pts. Life	
	How do you handle stress?
Living Situation	Are you successful in handling stress?
	Grooming/Hygiene
Additional Data:	

VALUE BELIEF PATTERN

Do you have any religious needs we should be aware of ?
What is important for us to know to give you good care?

Signature _____

Nursing the Aging: Opportunity and Challenge

Nursing Homes

Three levels of nursing care are provided in nursing home settings, and a facility may offer more than one level:

1. *Skilled nursing care* — for people who need 24-hour-a-day nursing care and supervision
2. *Supportive or intermediate care* — for those who are not able to live alone and require routine basic care, such as help with bathing and taking medications
3. *Residential or custodial care* — for those who need supervision and minimal help

The registered nurse usually functions in a leadership role, so there are unlimited opportunities for the licensed practical nurse to give hands-on care, follow through on procedures, and make patient assessments. In addition, the practical nurse may be given a position such as "charge nurse" after being instructed by and under the supervision of an R.N. (see the Job Description in this chapter).

The challenges of nursing home care will continue to increase due to early hospital discharge of more acutely ill older people and the addition of facilities for victims of Alzheimer's disease and AIDS.

In the Hospital

The hospital nurse is seeing more and more acutely ill older persons as medical, surgical, or hospice patients. Hospital nursing of aging patients demands these qualities:

1. Finely-tuned assessment skills
2. Technological know-how
3. The ability to assist with long-range planning for discharge in a minimal amount of time

Ethical issues are more complex in a hospital, and they are discussed in Chapter 1.

Home Health Care

Increasingly, the home health nurse is seeing older patients at retirement age living with family members or parents who are even older. These family members may be involved in the care of the patient and

Job Description

JOB TITLE: Charge Nurse   *DEPARTMENT:* Nursing

JOB SUMMARY: The charge nurse assumes responsibility for all the nursing care of patients on the unit to which he or she is assigned.

SUPERVISOR: Director of Nursing

RESPONSIBILITIES:

Patient Care Management:

- Knows all the patients on the unit by name and diagnosis and can describe their treatment.
- Recognizes significant changes in the condition of patients and takes necessary action.
- Makes daily rounds to all patients and evaluates their immediate physical condition.
- Supervises rehabilitation procedures, i.e., good body alignment and bed positioning, transfer activities with the use of the gait belt, range of motion, bowel and bladder training, decubitus and skin care.
- Prepares and administers medications and treatments as prescribed.
- Coordinates the care of the patient so that he/she receives the personal care, therapies, and recreation required within the limits of fatigue and patient interest.
- Has read the patients' rights and ensures that all staff and patients have read and understood them.
- Handles patient/guarantor complaints in a professional, conscientious manner and initiates any necessary corrective action.

Staff Management:

- Works with Patient Care Team to plan and meet the individual needs of each patient.
- Assigns unit personnel to patient care according to the patient's condition and the employee's level of competence.
- Supervises personnel to ensure care is given to patients.
- Completes annual employee evaluations.
- Encourages personnel to use 24 Hour Reality Orientation.

Records and Reports:

- Initiates nursing care plans and makes provision for updating each plan at least monthly.

Records and Reports (continued)

- Prepares and maintains inpatient records.
- Records pertinent facts about each patient in his medical records and writes a weekly summary showing progress or deterioration.
- Insures reports are made on all incidents.
- Keeps director of nursing informed of patient status and other matters pertinent to the unit through written reports and verbal communications.
- Meets with activity coordinator to promote good communications between nursing and activity.
- Obtains orders from physician, follows those orders, and reviews them and updates them on a monthly basis with the physician.
- Keeps physician informed of patient status changes.
- Gives and receives shift reports.

Department Management:

- Maintains a safe and clean environment.
- Establishes a cleaning schedule for utility rooms, nurses' station, and patients' closets and personal bedside equipment.
- Assigns duties from the cleaning schedule to staff and supervises their performance.
- Accompanies and assists physician during his patient rounds.
- Maintains drugs according to regulations.
- Attends staff programs as required.
- Attends regularly scheduled conferences with nurses, aides and orderlies on the unit to promote participation in planning patient care.
- Provides informal inservice as patient care needs dictate.
- Performs other duties as directed by the director of nursing.

Qualifications:

- Must be a graduate of an approved school of nursing or practical nursing and licensed to practice in this state.
- Must be willing to learn managerial skills and assume responsibility for a patient unit.
- Must be able to work a rotation of weekends and holidays.
- Must be able to communicate with people and cope with the emotions that surround the geriatric patient.
- Must wear appropriate uniforms and be neat and clean in appearance.

(Courtesy of Americana Healthcare Center, 600 S. Webster, Green Bay, WI.)

may be in need of care themselves. The home health care nurse deals with older people of all ages in the same residence. Home health care is an expanding field, and Chapter 10 discusses nursing responsibilities in this setting.

Gerontological Nurse Practitioners

The gerontological nurse practitioner practices independently, as a colleague with the physician, in hospitals, nursing homes, housing units, senior centers, community service centers, rehabilitation centers, and anywhere within a community where old people are clustered.

Functions of these nurses depend on the setting. In hospitals and nursing homes, nurse practitioners can do health assessments, preliminary physical examinations, and order diagnostic tests. Counseling, discharge planning, and in-service education are other responsibilities. Senior citizen housing units could employ gerontological nurse practitioners to provide primary health care and health maintenance for residents.

The Nurse As An Advocate

To be an advocate is to be supportive. In the hospital world of high technology, rapidly occurring events, and complicated Medicare forms, the elderly patient needs all the support he can get just to make it through the system. The nurse informs, counsels, and then supports the older person in making decisions and expressing needs. The independence of the older adult must be guarded and, whenever possible, the nurse should make situations convenient for patient and family without taking over. Any coordinating or planning, unless the elderly person is confused, should be a joint effort.

An advocate nurse monitors care. Conflict with the system or with the family is a possibility. When ethical and legal dilemmas result, the nurse should know the channels of communication to which she has access.

The nurse who is an advocate for the aged should consider joining a community organization that addresses issues of the older population. In an aging America, this is an opportunity for the nurse to influence her own future.

Summary

According to historical accounts, the care of sick older people was once the responsibility of families, religious orders, or poorly prepared caregivers in public hospitals. The development of the fields of geriatrics and gerontology in nursing was strengthened by the establishment in 1966 of the ANA Division of Gerontological Nursing, which set standards of practice, and placed an emphasis on wellness. The focus of nursing is on meeting basic needs through the nursing process. In nursing assessment of older persons, the nurse must be aware that, due to a lifetime of experiences, the older patient may not remember details that are necessary in preventing problems. Time and patience are required to obtain a history and identify stressors, and the input of significant others is crucial. A functional assessment will tell the nurse what the patient could do before he entered the hospital, and it is the baseline for discharge planning.

With the older population increasing, the hospital nurse is caring primarily for the acutely ill older person. Early discharge means nursing homes will need to offer more skilled nursing care and home health care agencies will increase in number. Keeping older people well will be a concern of these health care providers and the nurses they employ.

Activities

1. Interview nurse(s) who graduated before 1970 about their education in geriatric nursing.
2. Using the guidelines in this chapter, do a health history on an older person you know. How easy was it for you to get answers to questions? Were there things that the older person
   a. seemed reluctant to discuss?
   b. had forgotten?
   c. thought were unimportant?
3. What must the nurse ask and do in assessing the following patient:

   Mrs. A is 70 years old and has been in the hospital for two days with back pain. When the nurse removes her supper tray, Mrs. A states that her back pain is "spreading."

4. Visit a nursing home and ask about differences in the responsibilities of registered nurses and licensed practical nurses. Compare to Job Description at the end of this chapter.

Bibliography

Bullough V, Bullough B: The Care of the Sick. The Emergence of Modern Nursing. New York, Prodist, 1978

Burns N, Grove S: The Practice of Nursing Research. Conduct, Critique, and Utilization. Philadelphia, WB Saunders, 1987

Dakin F, Thompson E: Simplified Nursing, 5th ed. Philadelphia, JB Lippincott, 1951

Dolan J: Nursing in Society. A Historical Perspective, 14th ed. Philadelphia, WB Saunders, 1978

Fitzsimons VM: Maintaining a positive environment for the older adult. Orthop Nurs 4:48–51, 1985

Griffin G, Griffin J: History and Trends of Professional Nursing, 7th ed. St. Louis, CV Mosby, 1973

Hall G: Alterations in thought process. J Gerontol Nurs 14:30–37, 1988

Howell T: Our Advancing Years. London, Phoenix House, 1953

Iverson-Carpenter M: Impaired skin integrity. J Gerontol Nurs 14:25–29, 1988

Kruczek T: How hospitals hurt old people. RN 49:17–19, 1986

Meis M: Loneliness in the elderly. Orthop Nurs 4:63–66, 1985

Milde F: Impaired physical mobility. J Gerontol Nurs 14:20–24, 1988

Penn C: Promoting independence. J Gerontol Nurs 14:14–19, 1988

Rantz M et al: Nursing diagnosis in long-term care. Am J Nurs 85:916–917, 926, 1985

Sellow G, Nuesse C: A History of Nursing. St. Louis, CV Mosby, 1946

Wright S: Tearing down walls . . . a nurse specialist in the care of the elderly. Nurs Mirror 161:48–49, 1985

Yurick A, Spier B, Robb S, et al: The Aged Person and the Nursing Process, 2nd ed. Norwalk, CT, Appleton Century Crofts, 1984

3

Normal Aging

Learning Objectives

When you complete this chapter, you should be able to:

1. *Briefly define the nine theories of biological aging.*
2. *Discuss factors in psychological aging.*
3. *Explain the difference between the "disengagement" and "activity" theories of aging.*
4. *Identify signs of aging that appear as a person grows older.*
5. *List general changes in body tissue and functions that are common as the body ages.*
6. *Discuss the problems in describing mental aging.*

Aging is a normal process, a slowing of body functions as a result of biological changes. What does it mean psychologically and sociologically? Is there a spiritual definition of aging? The poet Robert Browning wrote this verse:

Grow old along with me,
The best is yet to be.

In his book, *Time Flies*, comedian Bill Cosby evaluates those famous lines: "On days when I need aspirin to get out of bed, Browning is clearly a minor poet; but he was an optimist and there is always comfort in his lines, no matter how much you ache." Browning's poem and Cosby's humor reflect some truths about normal aging. There is discomfort; there is hope.

Theories of normal aging have been advanced at the biological, psychological, and sociological levels. Biological theories deal with change at the cellular level and with physiological factors that affect the human organism as a whole. Psychological theories of aging discuss personality development. Sociological studies of aging investigate the roles of older people and their interaction with the rest of society.

The aging personality and the aging body cannot be separated from each other. Psychosocial changes, for instance, can be affected by sensory impairment. In normal aging, the physical imperfections of a lifetime may become more pronounced, resulting in physical or psychological discomfort. This is an individual phenomenon. A spiritual concept of aging relates to the overall viewpoint and response of an older person to aging. The natural changes of aging can be mistaken for disease processes. Knowledge of normal aging in all its aspects is the basis for assessment in nursing.

Theories of Normal Aging

The Search for Eternal Youth

Ancient history describes concoctions made from plant or animal parts that were supposed to grow hair, nails, and teeth or restore sexual energy. The ingestion of the ground testicles of some ferocious beasts was particularly noted for sexual rejuvenation. In some societies, old men indulged in sexual rituals with young "goddesses" in order to be rejuvenated.

The idea of a "fountain of youth" probably originated with some wishful thinker who imagined a connection between bubbling water and youthfulness. In the 12th century, a legend told about a powerful Christian king who lived in the Orient and possessed a fountain whose waters could restore youth. Explorers searched unsuccessfully for this king for three centuries. Ponce de Leon was looking for a fountain of youth when he discovered Florida in 1513. Baths of all kinds were thought to preserve youthful appearance. Royal European ladies sat in milk baths, unaware that milk would be better for their skin if they put it *inside* their bodies. Elixirs, potions, gadgets, and diets claiming to halt the aging process have always been available.

Biological Aging

Investigations in this century have yielded a number of theories about the biological process of aging. None of them is entirely right or wrong, and they all provide clues to the mystery. It is difficult to define universal factors about the mechanisms of aging. Humans do not all show the same changes at the same chronological age. Biological aging affects all body systems, but decline of function varies from organ to organ. Although the basic aging pattern in humans is the same everywhere, the rate of aging is affected by many factors, including genetics, the environment, and standards of living.

Genetic

Experiments on human cells in artificial cultures show that cells divide a limited number of times before they die. This suggests that every person inherits a program for his or her lifespan, called a "biological clock" or "genetic clock."

Another genetic theory states that when the body is no longer able to reproduce cells, then decline of the body follows.

Errors in Protein Synthesis

Protein synthesis, or production, plays a major role in the growth and reproduction of body cells, and it is the chief process of repair. Cells that are destroyed daily are replaced and wounds heal. The "error theory" states that mistakes in protein synthesis can occur and will disorganize cell function. As these errors are passed on, they collect over a period of time and cause changes — called aging — in organs and tissues. Errors in protein synthesis within the cell can be random or they can be introduced by other factors, such as radiation.

Immunological Dysfunctions

The immune system protects the body from foreign proteins, such as bacteria and viruses, by secreting antibodies to destroy them. What happens if cells change with age — could they be treated as foreign protein? That is one possibility.

Another possibility is that, with age, these antibodies cannot always distinguish between normal and abnormal proteins; they sometimes attack normal cells and cause damage or aging. A third possibility is that the white blood cells, lymphocytes, that produce the antibodies become less efficient.

Cross-linking

Connective tissue is abundant throughout the body. This tissue provides the framework that supports other tissues. The proteins in these tissues bond with one another, cross-linking, as one grows older. This causes the loss of elasticity in body organs and structures along with dryness and sagging of the skin.

Free Radicals

A free radical is a highly reactive chemical that has an extra electron. Free radicals are produced inside the body in the course of normal living by the oxidation of fats, carbohydrates, and proteins, and when oxygen combines with other substances in the cell, such as environmental pollutants. This chemical reacts with and damages normal cells when it accumulates in body cells faster than it can be eliminated.

Other Biological Theories of Aging

Lipofuscin is a by-product of metabolism with no known function. With age, particles of this yellow-brown pigment accumulate in body organs and structures and may disrupt normal cell metabolism.

There may be a connection between decreased endocrine function and growing old, because some hormone preparations reverse signs of aging. Those who view the body as a complicated machine believe that injury and overuse will wear it out. The theory that stress causes aging is popular with some because stress has many adverse effects on the body, such as precipitating heart attacks.

Psychological Theories of Aging

To age is to become a complete personality. The psychologist, Carl Jung, taught that one must accept death and reflect on the meaning of life in order to develop a healthy personality in old age. Other psychologists have offered theories on aging that identify stages one must pass through and the growth or learning that should occur in each stage. If this growth does not take place, a person can have problems that affect further development. For instance, if one does not learn to trust others at an early age, it may be difficult to do so later in life. According to theories of development by stages, old age is the time of life when one should feel that whatever has happened, life was worth living, and one is a valuable human being. One then goes on to adjust to normal changes, such as retirement and the loss of loved ones.

Sociological Theories of Aging

Sociological theories of aging describe how one's roles change as one grows older. The "disengagement theory" teaches that aging is a process in which older people gradually withdraw from life and responsibility and allow younger people to make decisions and to become leaders. The older person benefits by becoming free to relax and take time for himself. Critics of this theory point out that many older people do not wish to withdraw from responsible roles and that improved health care and living conditions in the future will further discourage them from doing so.

The "activity theory," in contrast to the disengagement theory, maintains that one should deny old age as long as possible. The positive aspect of this theory is that an active life-style that uses body, mind, and common sense contributes to health and well-being. The truth, however, is that not all older people want to stay young, nor do they possess the health and capabilities necessary to "postpone" old age.

Aging As Spiritual Development

There are hints about spiritual development as a definition of aging in some of the psychological theories, for instance in discussions of a meaning for existence. Leo Buscaglia, educator, writer, and lecturer on the subject of love and relationships, has a theory on personality development that discusses the mature person's relationship with God. In his description of the fully functioning old person, Buscaglia discusses inner resources and the emergence of the "true self."

Anthropologist and social biologist Ashley Montagu describes a progression of "goodness" in personality development that might be considered spiritual.

Theories of aging as spiritual development, more than any other aging theory, look at aging as an individual matter. Here is one spiritual definition of aging as a normal process: Aging is a winding down of the body and a spiraling up of the mind and soul. Physical capabilities diminish so that one can eventually sit still. It becomes harder to see and hear the distractions of the world so that one can focus on the internal environment of values, beliefs, and feelings. The outcome of this process is determined by how one adapts to the reality of approaching death. In this respect, aging as a spiritual process is controlled by the individual. When one accepts death as natural and normal, it is possible to find an answer to the universal question, "Who and why am I?"

Normal Physical Aging

Aging Anatomy

Aging produces changes in human anatomy and physiology that predispose older people to health problems. Chapter 6 discusses common problems of normal aging with nursing implications.

Height and Posture

People get shorter with age, but not only because of changes in their bones and muscles. Statistics show that people, in general, are becoming taller with each successive generation. The effects of illness, amount of physical activity, nutrition, and race are not completely understood.

The aged person is somewhat stooped in appearance and this makes the extremities look longer. Actually, bone is reabsorbed from the inside surface of the long bones faster than it is formed on the outside surfaces, but this does not affect length. In a very old person, the extremities only appear longer because the spinal column is shorter, accounting for loss of height. The fibrocartilage intervertebral discs become drier and thinner. With increasing age, bone decreases in mass and mineral content and the vertebrae compress into shorter, wider structures (Fig. 3–1). A decline in estrogen production in the aging female accelerates the loss of calcium from the bone, causing osteoporosis.

Height is affected by varying degrees of thoracic kyphosis, a curvature of the spine known as "humpback." The pelvis widens and a slight flexion of hips and knees also decrease stature. Loss of muscle strength and muscle mass add to the stooped, forward-leaning posture and flexion of the lower extremities.

To compensate for the spinal curve, the neck is tilted back and held in extension to keep the head up. The extensor muscles of the neck become thicker and the anterior flexor muscles of the neck atrophy and become shorter. The scapulae, or shoulder blades, move forward with the curve and the shoulder span narrows. The lower back becomes flat.

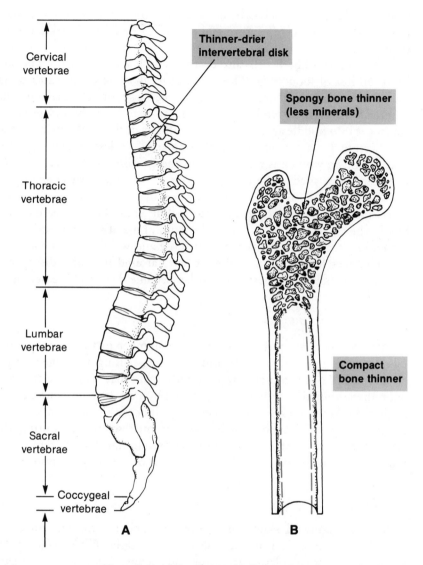

Cervical vertebrae

Thinner-drier intervertebral disk

Spongy bone thinner (less minerals)

Thoracic vertebrae

Lumbar vertebrae

Sacral vertebrae

Coccygeal vertebrae

Compact bone thinner

A

B

Figure 3–1. Aging changes in the bones.

Water, Fat, and Body Weight

Ancient researchers believed that aging was related to water loss and the drying out of the body. They were not entirely wrong. With age there is a decrease both in intracellular and extracellular fluids, and this is one of the reasons dehydration occurs rapidly in the elderly. The composition of electrolytes, acids, bases, and salts that control cell activities remains the same. Temperature and acidity of body fluids remain constant from youth to old age.

The number of body cells also decreases with age. By age 65, a person has a cell loss of about 30%. This does not mean a one-third reduction in size. Body fat accumulates with age and the large fat cells make up the difference in mass. Overall body weight increases slowly and peaks as adults get into middle age, and then it gradually declines. Women tend to gain weight for a longer period of time and lose less as they age. Fat distribution in women is mostly on the chest, waist, hips, and thighs. In men, fat is deposited at the waist and over the chest and lower abdomen.

With very old age there is a decrease in subcutaneous fat in both sexes, predisposing elderly persons to feeling cold. The decrease occurs first in the extremities and then in the trunk. Loss of subcutaneous fat in the extremities makes the skin appear loose and wrinkled over the muscle. The eyes look sunken as the fat layer around the orbit disappears. Hollows in shoulders, chest, and axillae become deep and breasts sag.

Muscle Mass and Strength

Muscle fibers atrophy and decrease in number in the aging person. Fibrous tissue gradually replaces muscle tissue, causing a decline in muscle strength. Loss of muscle strength with aging may also be related to a poor dietary intake of potassium, as well as to loss of neurons and hormones. Aging muscle does not work well because it is not as efficient in using oxygen. Tendons shrink and become sclerotic, limiting the strength and range of movement of the extremities. Slight tremors are normal and are associated with degeneration of the nervous system.

Skin and Accessory Organs

Normal aging of skin is influenced by diet, health, exposure, and heredity. Skin dries and the outer layer turns fragile. The collagen fibers in the dermis, or vascular layer, shrink and become rigid, making the skin less elastic. The loss of subcutaneous fat results in lines, wrinkles, and sagging. Pigment cells—melanocytes—gather and cause age spots.

A decrease in melanin, the color pigment, in hair follicles produces graying of hair. Hair loss occurs more prominently in men. Overall body hair diminishes as one gets older. Scalp, pubic, and axillary hair thins. However, hair in the nose and ears gets thicker, and a woman may note the beginning of a mustache.

Nails of the fingers and toes grow more slowly, turning hard and brittle with long bumpy stripes. The sudoriferous, or sweat, glands diminish in number, size, and activity as they become fibrotic. Older persons are more susceptible to heat stroke. Sebaceous glands secrete less oil to lubricate hair and skin, and dryness is the result.

Aging of Systems and Organs

Cardiovascular System (Fig. 3–2)

In the aging heart, the most common change is in the myocardium, the thick layer of muscle. Lipofuscin pigment, a by-product of metabolism, collects and gives the heart a brown color. Muscle fibers decrease and some are replaced by fibrous tissue. Oxygen is used less efficiently.

Four sets of heart valves permit the flow of blood from the atria or upper chambers of the heart into the lower chambers or ventricles and

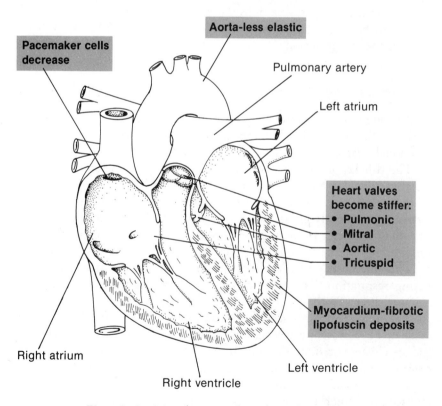

Figure 3–2. Aging changes in the cardiovascular system.

from the ventricles into the aorta and pulmonary artery. With age these valves stiffen and become thicker as the collagen degenerates and fat accumulates. The pacemaker cells in the wall of the right atrium that cause the heart muscle to contract and relax decrease in number. Pulse irregularities are common in the aging.

Cardiac output, the amount of blood pumped into the aorta and the pulmonary artery during each beat, decreases by 25% in the older person. The aorta and other large arteries are less elastic with age. This is arteriosclerosis, a hardening of the arteries due to localized accumulations of fat. It has been said that a man is only as old as his arteries. Blood vessels, in general, are less elastic; they accumulate calcium deposits and become narrower. Peripheral blood flow, the circulation in the extremities, meets more resistance. Blood flow through the kidneys is decreased. A rise in blood pressure is associated with changes of aging. Heredity, diet, and disease are factors that contribute to the aging of the heart.

Under normal, nonstressful conditions, the older person's heart will adapt well to its functional ability. When more is demanded of it—for instance, when that person climbs stairs or shovels snow—the heart will respond by beating too rapidly. It takes longer for the heart to slow down again in the aging person.

Respiratory System (Fig. 3-3)

Although the respiratory system includes the nose, throat, and trachea, it is the thorax and the lungs that undergo the major structural and functional changes of aging.

The thorax, or rib cage, is formed by the sternum or breastbone, the costal cartilages which connect the ribs with the sternum or with each other, the ribs, and the bodies of the thoracic vertebrae. Although costal cartilage is normally elastic, with age it becomes rigid and may calcify. The chest diameter from anterior to posterior increases, due to kyphosis, and a barrel-chest deformity may result.

The intercostal muscles help the diaphragm move the chest wall during respiration. These muscles fill the spaces between the ribs and connect them. With age, the intercostals atrophy and become weaker.

The lungs are composed of a porous, spongy substance. Each lung is made up of microscopic cavities called alveoli. Alveoli are covered by sacs and are clustered around the tiny tubes—alveolar ducts—that branch off from the bronchi, which bring the air to the lungs. The alveoli have fragile membranes and contain capillaries. An alveolar duct with its sacs looks like a bunch of grapes. It is estimated that there are 300 million alveoli in the lungs. The amount of surface area this adds up to is

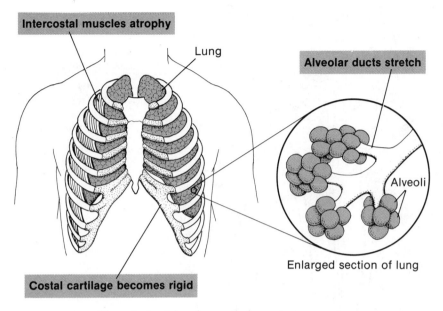

Intercostal muscles atrophy

Lung

Alveolar ducts stretch

Alveoli

Enlarged section of lung

Costal cartilage becomes rigid

Figure 3–3. Aging changes in the respiratory system.

enormous. Loss of elasticity in the tissue causes the alveolar ducts and the alveoli to become stretched.

These changes in the lungs and thorax mean decreased lung expansion. When the older person takes a breath, the bases of the lungs do not inflate well and secretions that collect in the lungs are not expelled. The residual volume is the amount of air that stays in the lungs after exhalation. The older person exhales incompletely and the residual volume increases. This, in turn, reduces vital capacity, which is the largest amount of air that can be forcibly expelled following the deepest inspiration. As parts of the lung remain underventilated, the blood coming into the lungs may be poorly oxygenated. The older person is at high risk for pneumonia.

Dental System *(Fig. 3–4)*

The extent of tooth loss is influenced by diet, jaw structure, other teeth, the mechanics of chewing, oral hygiene, and professional care. Becoming edentulous, or toothless, is *not* inevitable in the aging process.

The enamel covering of the teeth becomes thinner over a lifetime, and teeth become darker as the dentin, which is the body of the tooth, shows through. Repeated contact with substances that stain also make the

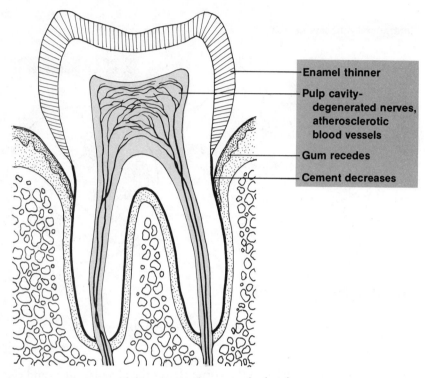

Enamel thinner

Pulp cavity-
degenerated nerves,
atherosclerotic
blood vessels

Gum recedes

Cement decreases

Figure 3–4. Aging changes in the dental system.

enamel darker. Odontoblasts, the cells that produce dentin, change and diminish with time. Degeneration of nerves and atherosclerosis of blood vessels take place in the pulp cavity. The cement that holds the tooth in place decreases with age and is exposed as gums recede (see Fig. 3-4). Receding gums deprive the cement of nourishment. Fat deposits and fibrosis in the salivary glands reduce secretions and the whole mouth becomes dry.

Digestive System *(Fig. 3–5)*

The esophagus is the muscular tube from the throat to the stomach. It has sphincters at each end that remain closed until food is swallowed. Peristalsis is the wavelike movement along the muscles of the gastrointestinal tract that moves food through the system. Peristalsis begins in the esophagus and it affects the opening and closing of the sphincters. As a person ages, peristaltic contractions in the esophagus decrease and interfere with the passage of food into the stomach and the proper functioning

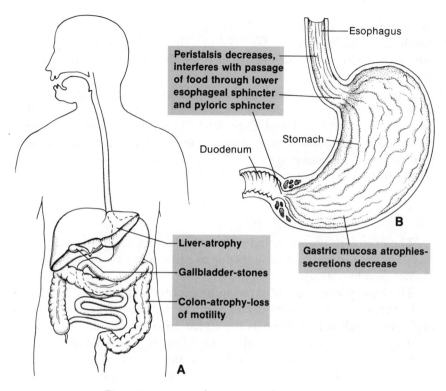

Esophagus

Peristalsis decreases, interferes with passage of food through lower esophageal sphincter and pyloric sphincter

Stomach

Duodenum

B

Liver-atrophy

Gallbladder-stones

Colon-atrophy-loss of motility

Gastric mucosa atrophies- secretions decrease

A

Figure 3–5. Aging changes in the digestive system.

of the sphincters. Other contractions of the muscle occur and they, too, interfere with the movement of food.

The mucous lining of the stomach — gastric mucosa — is normally thick with glands that secrete acid, mucin, and enzymes. With age, the gastric mucosa atrophies and secretions diminish. It is unclear whether or not movements of the stomach are affected by age.

Villi are minute, finger-like projections on the mucous membrane lining the small intestine. They number between four and five million, and each one contains a lymph channel and a network of capillaries. Around the villi are cells with microvilli. Digested food is absorbed into both. Because of the large number of these tiny projections, the surface area of the small intestine is about ten square miles. A decrease in cells and enzymes due to aging, therefore, does not greatly affect absorption in the small intestine. Peristalsis is decreased. In the colon, or large intestine, where the electrolytes and water are absorbed from the indigestible components of food, there is also some atrophy and reduced motility.

The liver gets smaller with age, decreasing the space it has to store blood, minerals, and vitamins. Liver functions of synthesizing bile and metabolizing carbohydrates, fats, and proteins are basically unaltered by age alone. Changes in enzymes reduce the liver's ability to metabolize drugs.

The gallbladder, a pear-shaped sac under the liver, is a reservoir for the bile, which it expels into the small intestine when stimulated by the presence of gastric acid and fatty food. The incidence of gallstones, consisting mainly of cholesterol, protein, and the pigment bilirubin, does increase with advancing age. The formation of gallstones seems to be related to bile that is high in cholesterol.

Excretory System *(Fig. 3–6)*

The excretory system includes the kidneys, ureters, bladder, and urethra. The most significant changes due to aging occur in the kidneys and bladder (see Fig. 3–6).

The kidney loses weight in the aging process—as much as 20%. As a result there is about a 30% decrease in the number of nephrons. The nephron, which makes urine, is the functioning unit of the kidney. At birth a person has about one million nephrons in each kidney.

A nephron consists of a glomerulus, which is a cluster of capillaries partially enclosed in a capsule called Bowman's capsule, its tubule, and a

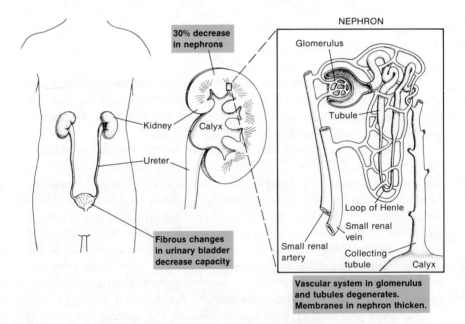

Figure 3–6. *Aging changes in the nephron.*

blood supply (Fig. 3–6). Filtration takes place from the blood in the glomeruli into the Bowman's capsules. The tubules extend from the capsules and, by various mechanisms, they reabsorb the substances needed by the body; they also excrete water and waste substances.

Thickening of membranes in the nephrons and degeneration in the vascular system occur with age. The rates of filtration, excretion, and reabsorption decline. This affects the amount of a drug that is reabsorbed or excreted and helps account for problems older people have with medications. Blood flow to the kidney is decreased. Formation of urine is lower in the aging kidney, but the filtration process remains efficient, keeping the acid–base balance stable in the body.

The bladder is a collapsible muscular bag lined with a mucous membrane; it stores urine. Fibrous changes in the lining and weakened muscles can be attributed to aging. Capacity for holding urine is decreased. The reflex that brings about contraction of the bladder muscles and relaxation of the internal sphincter to begin the urinating process is delayed.

Reproductive System

In the female, the aging process accelerates with menopause due to hormonal changes. As the ovaries cease to function, that is, to develop ova and secrete hormones, they gradually become smaller, sclerotic, and rolled up (Fig. 3–7). The fallopian tubes atrophy and become shorter.

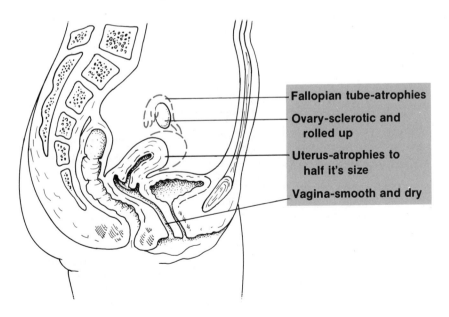

Figure 3–7. Aging changes in the female reproductive system.

The greatest atrophy takes place in the uterus, which becomes the size it was before puberty. In the endometrium, the inner lining that serves as a "nest" for a developing baby and sloughs off during menstruation, cells become fibrous and cystic. The myometrium, a thick muscular layer, also becomes fibrotic. Blood vessels throughout the uterus thicken with sclerotic changes.

In the vagina, the surface layer of the mucous membrane becomes thin and avascular. Loss of elastic tissue and secretions makes the older vagina look pink, smooth, and dry. The vagina is more alkaline in older females. Externally, the genitalia appear flattened and wrinkled due to loss of subcutaneous tissue and to vascular changes, and pubic hair is thinner.

In the male, the prostate gland circles the urethra just below the bladder. Normally it is the shape and size of a chestnut. It secretes seminal fluid that protects sperm. As a man ages, this gland enlarges with cell overgrowth (hyperplasia) and it may constrict the urethra (Fig. 3–8). Prostatic hypertrophy causes difficulty in urinating.

The male testes, located in the scrotum, produce sperm and secrete hormones. With age these glands become smaller and firmer, and sperm production is decreased. Tissue and vascular changes affect the structure of the external male genitalia, which includes the scrotum and the penis. Fibrous tissue encroaches upon muscle, and blood vessels become sclerotic.

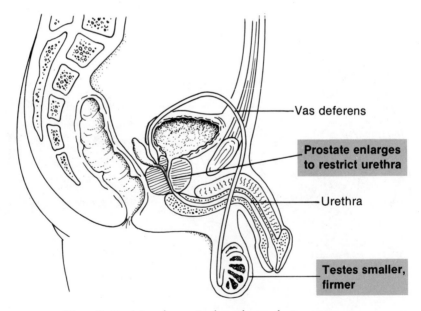

Figure 3–8. *Aging changes in the male reproductive system.*

Endocrine System

The endocrine system is made up of glands that secrete hormones directly into the bloodstream. However, hormonal secretion of two of the glands associated with this system, the pineal and the thymus, is debatable. The metabolic functions of the body and the rates of chemical reactions in the cells are regulated by the endocrine system. The scope and complexity of the endocrine system are better understood by an overall look at its components and the effects of aging insofar as they are known (Table 3–1).

Nervous System

The brain, the spinal cord, and the nerves are the components of the nervous system. The nervous system organizes body functions by regulating activities such as skeletal movements, smooth muscle contractions, and numerous glandular secretions. Communication from one part of the body to another is a major task in this organization process.

Since the nervous system is affected by all other systems, it is difficult to identify specific changes due to aging. In general, there is a reduction of neurons, decreased blood flow to the brain and reduced metabolism.

Gradual thickening and fibrosis of the dura mater, arachnoid, and pia mater (the coverings of the brain) occur (Fig. 3–9). The brain atrophies and the pigment, lipofuscin, can be identified in the gray matter. More fat can also be seen in an aged brain. Microscopically, there is increased branching of fibrils from cells and there is some cell hypertrophy. Decreased vascularity and fibrotic changes in the spinal cord and nerves are similar to those in the brain.

Sensory Organs

Aging reduces the efficiency of the five senses: sight, hearing, touch, smell, and taste. Vision probably undergoes the most significant changes.

The eyeball, the optic nerve, and the accessory organs around the eye are the parts of the visual system (Fig. 3–10). With advancing age, loss of orbital fat can cause backward displacement of the eye and drooping of the eyelids. The secretions of the lacrimal (tear) ducts are diminished and the eye looks dry or dull. Reduced elasticity in the eye muscles and lens capsule affects the focusing power of the eye, resulting in presbyopia, or farsightedness, which may begin in middle age. Peripheral vision is difficult as the visual field narrows.

The deposition of fat on the edge of the cornea produces a white circle around the iris, called arcus senilis. The pupil is smaller, which may

Table 3–1. The Endocrine System and Aging

Name	Location	Function	Aging Changes
Pineal	Attached to posterior part of third ventricle of brain	High metabolic function; hormone?	Degenerates early in life
Pituitary (Hypophysis, two glands)	Sella turcica of sphenoid bone	Two glands secrete total of nine hormones affecting growth and functions of other glands and organs	Decreased secretion; significance unknown
Thyroid	Neck, just below larynx	Secretes two hormones to regulate metabolic rate and processes of growth and tissue differentiation	Decreased secretion; nodular formation; decreased metabolic rate; Thin hair, dry skin
Parathyroid (two or more)	Attached to posterior thyroid	Secretes hormone to maintain homeostasis of blood calcium level	Probably none
Thymus	In chest, below thyroid	Secretes hormone that enables lymphocytes to convert to plasma cells?	Atrophies gradually
Isles of Langerhans (Pancreas)	Behind stomach	Secrete insulin, glucogen; affect metabolism and particularly blood sugar	Decreased secretions; decreased ability to metabolize glucose
Adrenals (two)	One on top of each kidney	Secrete hormones to help with normal metabolism, growth of bones and reproductive system; help body resist stress	Decreased secretions; significance unclear
Ovaries (two)	Lower abdomen	Secrete sex hormones to affect reproduction and growth	See changes described under reproductive system
Testes (two)	Scrotum	Secrete sex hormone to aid in development of secondary sex characteristics	See changes described under reproductive system

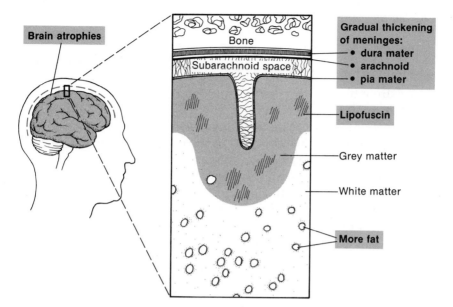

Brain atrophies

Bone

Gradual thickening
of meninges:
● dura mater
● arachnoid
● pia mater

Subarachnoid space

Lipofuscin

Grey matter

White matter

More fat

Figure 3-9. Aging changes in the brain.

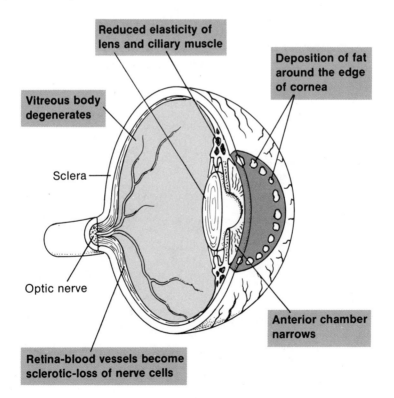

Reduced elasticity of
lens and ciliary muscle

Deposition of fat
around the edge
of cornea

Vitreous body
degenerates

Sclera

Optic nerve

Anterior chamber
narrows

Retina-blood vessels become
sclerotic-loss of nerve cells

Figure 3-10. Aging changes in the eye.

be due to increased rigidity and atrophy of the iris. A shallow anterior chamber is common in the aging eye. The aqueous humor is formed in the eye from blood in the capillaries and drains out again through small veins at a consistent rate to maintain a constant intraocular pressure. With aging, this system is not as efficient and intraocular pressure may rise, increasing the risk of glaucoma. Yellowing of the lens alters color perception. Progressive degeneration of the vitreous body, the soft gelatinous substance in the eyeball, can result in opaque particles or "floaters" appearing in one's vision. Blood vessels get sclerotic in the retina, where visual images are transmitted to the brain, and there also may be a loss of nerve cells in this area. Night vision is impaired.

The hearing apparatus is made up of the ears, the auditory nerves, and the auditory areas of the temporal lobes of the cerebrum. In the ear, certain conditions can be identified and related to advancing age. These occur in the middle ear and in the structures of the inner ear (Fig. 3–11). The tympanic membrane (eardrum) thickens and loses its elasticity. The ossicular chain, three tiny movable bones — the malleus or hammer, incus or anvil, and the stapes or stirrups — are located on the inner side of the tympanic membrane in the middle ear. These bones receive the vibrations of the tympanic membrane , magnify them, and pass them on to the inner ear. The efficiency of these bones is lost when the tympanic membrane loses some of its function; conduction deafness may result.

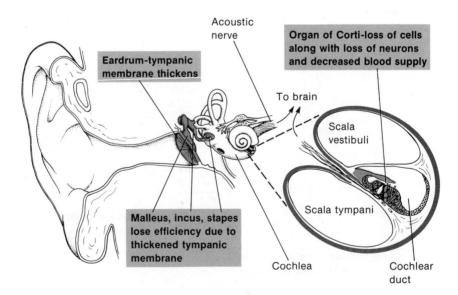

Figure 3–11. Aging changes in the ear.

The inner ear collects the vibrations of a sound, passes it through its system to the organ of Corti, which lies along the length of the cochlear duct, and sends impulses to the brain. The organ of Corti consists of supportive cells and hair cells, which are topped with a membrane. Nerve cells begin at the base of the hair cells. The movement of the hair cells against this membrane stimulates the dendrites, the projections of the nerve cells, and initiates impulse conduction by the cochlear nerve to the brainstem. Changes in this mechanism due to aging include loss of hair cells and supportive cells in the organ of Corti, loss of neurons in the cochlea and auditory pathways, atrophy, and loss of blood supply.

All of these conditions contribute to a progressive loss of hearing as one grows older that is known as "presbycusis." Change is gradual and is accompanied by functional abnormalities:

- Impaired sensitivity, especially to higher sounds
- Loss of directional hearing, inability to locate sound
- Abnormal perception of loudness, may be hypersensitive
- Difficulty in discrimination between sounds, especially in speech
- Tinnitus, a ringing in the ears
- Decline in the ability to process sound

Accumulation of cerumen, or wax, in the ears of the elderly is common enough to be considered age-related and impairs hearing. Maintenance of equilibrium is part of inner ear function. The prevalence of vertigo increases with age and may be due to degeneration of this structure.

Taste buds are reduced and become less efficient with age. The sense of smell decreases also. Tactile sensation, sense of touch, also decreases with loss of neurons and vascular and tissue changes.

Memory, Intelligence, and Learning

Alteration of memory is common in normal aging. Short-term memory loss may occur, while memory remains keen for events long past. Measuring intelligence in older people is of limited value because contributing factors such as different educational backgrounds and health deficits may affect a test's accuracy. The number of brilliant and productive older people always in evidence should lead one to the conclusion that intelligence does not decline with age. Older people possess individual capacities for learning that are influenced by other factors, such as motivation and readiness, just as they are in younger people. Learning motor skills may be more difficult in old age because of physiological changes. More time may be required to learn new habits because an older person has had a long time to practice existing habits. An older person may also need more time to begin a new learning experience.

Normal Aging

Old age is a unique experience for everyone who achieves it. It is the stage of life when all the little physical imperfections one has noted through the years may become more pronounced. Aging muscles and ligaments cause the body to sag and, when a person is lying down, this puts pressure on blood vessels and nerves, with the result that limbs become numb or painful and often wake one out of sound sleep. Foot bones that were never perfect grow more knobs and allow bunions and corns to flourish. Varicose veins that existed for years become more prominent. Normal aging is always accompanied by changes in body structure and function.

A Philosophical Viewpoint for Nurses

A nurse of any age is well advised to remember that normal aging is often uncomfortable and inconvenient, but it is not a disease. Older people are well aware of the time and patience it requires to care for them or to help them help themselves. A nurse of any age is approaching old age, but he or she will not reach it any sooner by close contact with, and caring for, old people. During a Gray Panther function on the Atlantic City boardwalk, Maggie Kuhn wore a sign that said, "Touch me, wrinkles are not contagious."

A sense of humor and a sense of the divine are worth cultivating in order to keep the process of normal aging in proper perspective (see "The Best is Yet to Come").

The Best is Yet to Come

Though I am growing old, I maintain that the best part is yet to come — the time when one may see things more dispassionately and know oneself and others more truly, and perhaps be able to do more, and in religion rest centered in a few simple truths. I do not want to ignore the other side, that one will not be able to see so well or walk so far or read so much. But there may be more peace within more communion with God, more real light instead of distraction about many things, better relations with others, fewer mistakes.

Benjamin Jowett, 19th century British classical scholar

Summary

Throughout recorded history there are accounts of people's search for eternal youth. The fact is that we grow old, and we do so at varying rates. There are many theories about why and how the aging process takes place. Biological theories discuss errors in cell formation and decreased function within cells. There are theories that the body ages from stress and that the body simply wears out from use. Psychological theories describe changes in personality development, and sociologists study the changing roles of older people in society. The spiritual response to aging may include acceptance of growing old and a mature meditation on life's meaning.

In normal aging, systems slow down due to changes in body structures. Tissues become inelastic, thicker, or thinner. Secretions, in many instances, decrease or change in character. Bones become thinner and neurons decrease. With a decrease in number of neurons, older people have slower reaction times. Intelligence does not diminish with age, although there may be alterations in memory.

Activities

1. If you could choose between the "disengagement" and "activity" theories of aging, which would you prefer, and why?
2. Select one theory of aging (biological, psychological, sociological, or spiritual), and list ways it could affect nursing care.
3. Trace a sound wave through an aging ear. Describe possible problems.
4. Write four general, positive statements about normal aging.
5. In the following list of conditions, *circle* those that occur as a *normal* part of the aging process:

Glaucoma	Enlarged heart
Being senile	Slower heart rate
Slower kidneys	Less feeling of hot and cold on
Heart attacks	skin
Anxiety	Fewer sweat glands
Hardening of the arteries	Smaller taste buds
Reminiscing about the past	Loss of muscle tone
High blood pressure	Depression
Varicose veins	Long-term memory loss
Waking up at night	Short-term memory loss
Dry skin	Slower reaction time
More saliva	

Bibliography

Barash D: Aging. An Exploration. Seattle, University of Washington Press, 1983

Burnside I: Nursing and the Aged. A Self-Care Approach, 3rd ed. New York, McGraw-Hill, 1988

Ebersole P, Hess P: Toward Healthy Aging. Human Needs and Nursing Response, 2nd ed. St. Louis, CV Mosby, 1985

Eliopoulos C: Gerontological Nursing, 2nd ed. Philadelphia, JB Lippincott, 1987

Gress L, Bahr Sr R: The Aging Person. A Holistic Perspective. St. Louis, CV Mosby, 1984

Memmler R, Wood D: The Human Body in Health and Disease, 6th ed. Philadelphia, JB Lippincott, 1987

Pifer A, Bronte L (eds): Our Aging Society, Paradox and Promise. New York, WW Norton and Co, 1986

Rosdahl C: Textbook of Basic Nursing, 4th ed. Philadelphia, JB Lippincott, 1985

Rossman I: Clinical Geriatrics, 3rd ed. Philadelphia, JB Lippincott, 1987

Communicating with the Aging Person

Learning Objectives

When you complete this chapter, you should be able to:

1. Describe the communication process.
2. Identify guidelines for good listening.
3. Give an example of each of these communication skills:
   a. Reflective response
   b. Clarification
   c. An open question
4. Discuss barriers to communication that are related to age.
5. Describe the various kinds of nonverbal communication
6. List seven general blocks to communication.
7. Role-play a conversation with a person who is hard of hearing. What communication skills are especially important in this situation?
8. Write a paragraph on how to communicate with a confused older patient.
9. State four purposes of a health assessment interview.

When aging is not understood or is unacceptable, there is a tendency to talk *at* older persons or *around* them, rather than *to* them. If we think older persons cannot hear us or understand what we are saying, we talk as if they were not even present. Nurses and doctors are frequently guilty of this when they are in an older patient's room. A discussion of the patient's condition takes place across the bed, like this:

Doctor: "How did she sleep last night?"
Nurse: "She was restless."
Doctor: "Maybe we'll get her out of bed more today . . . "

Sometimes this is done with good intentions, but the result is no communication at all with the older person, and a less effective resolution of the problem under discussion.

Communication is the process by which we accept or reject any human being, condition, or event. Communication enables us to influence another person's behavior for better or for worse.

Although there are individual ways in which older people or those who interact with them set up their own communication blocks, there is no doubt that the age differences between people can be a natural barrier. Sincerity and awareness of the aging person as an individual with whom one shares human needs for personal contact and common bonds are the foundation of a trusting relationship and good communication (Fig. 4–1).

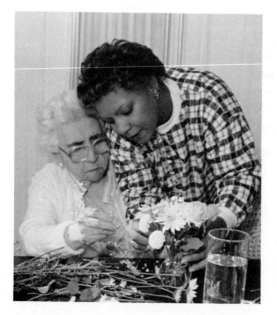

Figure 4–1. Good listening and sincere interest in an older person can overcome the communication barrier that age difference sometimes creates.

Communication: Its Definition and Importance to Nursing

Communication is the sending and receiving of messages in a two-way process. Messages are conveyed in words, actions, attitudes, and feelings. For this reason, communication is both "verbal" and "nonverbal." To communicate, one must have communication skills: one must know how to listen, observe, respond, and act. The conditions under which one communicates are also significant. This includes the place, the time, the space between communicators, and the limitations of the individuals. In this discussion, those limitations are due to aging and illness. Effective communication in nursing is often called "therapeutic" because it is helpful in achieving goals and promoting wellness. Therefore, effective communication is a major component of nursing. Interviewing, teaching, and interpreting are only some of the ways in which a nurse communicates with others. Every hands-on procedure, every touch, and every gesture can convey the message, "I care about you" or "This is only a job."

Listening and Understanding Older People

"Nobody Listens to Me!"

The great human desire is to be listened to and understood, and it goes largely unfulfilled. "Nobody listens to me!" is a universal cry. Seventy or eighty years of not being attentively listened to may be one reason why an older person is sometimes reluctant to talk or responds inappropriately to the nurse. One possible translation of "Why do you want to know *that*?" or "Nobody's bothered about that *before*," could be, "I've been telling people that for years and nobody paid any attention." "Nobody listens" implies that nobody cares. Effective communication begins with caring and becoming a good listener.

Unfortunately for the listening process, the brain works much faster than the average person speaks, giving the brain time to wander, engage in intuitive speculation, and jump to conclusions. Listening is a skill that is developed by practice and concentration.

What Is Good Listening?

Listening for *what needs to be heard* before responding to and initiating further communication is good listening. In communicating with an older person, the nurse must listen carefully to identify the central idea of what the older person is attempting to *say* or *ask*, his thoughts about it, and his feelings. In other words, listen for what *is* being said, or left unsaid, on a particular subject.

CASE STUDY

An 80-year-old man is having his blood pressure checked at a wellness clinic. He asks the nurse, "Do you know anything about getting those contraptions to wear around your neck to call for help? My daughter says I should have one." What is he asking?

Does this man want a description of an electronic unit in current use by old people living alone? The word "contraption" implies an unknown, or even something that arouses suspicion. He has not said the idea is his, so how does he feel about it? Does he also want to talk about his health? What has the nurse *heard*? Here is an aging man who evidently lives alone and may or may not feel safe in his independence. He needs information and reassurance about a device that will increase his safety. Perhaps he needs advice about health maintenance that is not related to his question.

Guidelines for Listening

Remain Quiet

To listen, first of all, one must remain quiet. Exceptions to this are when affirmation ("I see") or encouragement ("And then . . . ") is indicated. This seems obvious, yet it can be very difficult to keep silent, especially in a helping relationship where one wants to offer advice where advice appears warranted.

More difficulty arises because older people need time to process what they hear and then respond. Short-term memory deficits, confusion, or disorientation may prolong a dialogue. Restraint is often necessary when it seems that communication with the older person would be helped if the nurse finished a statement or a question. Such help proves to be no help at all because it implies that the speaker can't or doesn't know what he wants to say. The nurse's conclusion may be false and the older person's train of thought is disrupted. Any problem he may have with comprehension is magnified. Older people may allow themselves to be interrupted because they are often keenly aware of how long it takes them to say something. They may be distressed at having to command so much of someone else's time, especially when that someone is the nurse who is "so busy." The nurse must allow ample time for an older person to answer questions and to give information.

Establish Eye Contact

In listening, attention should remain focused on the speaker. The nurse should be relaxed and calm. Eye contact should be used as much as possible because it will make the speaker feel that what he has to say is important. Thick lenses in an older person's eyeglasses can make it hard to maintain eye contact, but the nurse should be willing to make the extra effort required to listen.

Avoid Distractions

Communicating in an environment where there are no distractions is not always possible. Ringing telephones and other background noises may be unavoidable. Minor actions by the nurses are distracting and they are often done unconsciously. They include snapping a rubber band, tapping a pencil or paper clip, shuffling paper, and twirling the end of a stethoscope. The nurse who is chewing gum makes it difficult for the older person who is attempting to read her lips while she speaks. Besides being distracted, the older patient may interpret these behaviors as signs of disinterest or impatience.

Empathize

To empathize is to put oneself in someone else's place, to see the situation from their viewpoint and to offer understanding. When that someone else is 50 years older, this is a real challenge. Older patients, unless they are confused, can distinguish empathy from apathy, and they can recognize when they are being humored rather than heard. They know a young nurse does not truly know how they feel. Sensitive listening, with attention to the details of maintaining eye contact, an open mind, and a positive attitude, will convince the older speaker that the nurse is making an honest effort to understand.

Separate Emotions and Feelings from the Listening Process

Emotions prevent one from hearing and understanding what is being *said.* The nurse who is overwhelmed by sadness, anger, or frustration cannot listen objectively. When we like a person, we are more likely to hear what they are saying and to be receptive to their ideas. Certainly there are patients to whom the nurse will be more drawn than others. Separating feelings about patients from the messages they are trying to give can be difficult. Learn to listen without being prejudiced by emotions and feelings in order to respond appropriately and to further communication.

Interpret Carefully

Remember that not all people use words the same way or think alike. Facts must be distinguished from what you *think* you have heard.

Show Respect

Attentive listening based on the preceding guidelines will help demonstrate respect for what the older person is saying. When the nurse shows this respect, that person feels valued and communication is open and honest.

What about the nurse who becomes bored with careful listening? Everyone becomes boring to listen to at some point, and any age difference between persons can be a factor: forty can be bored by twenty, and thirty by ten, twenty by fifteen, and the feelings are mutual. By their own admission, older people are prone to bore others by talking too much about the "good old days" to people who are younger than they are. In the good old days, they felt better, looked better, and had more fun — and those days are easier to remember in detail than the events of last summer. As one grows older, one may share fewer interests with those people one sees most often. Aches, pains, and chronic illness may be a major part of life, and so they are focal points of conversations. Although the tendency to moralize is not limited to any age group but is more dependent on personality, many older people moralize to a significant degree (perhaps because they know more and feel they have less to lose). On the other hand, they are full of wisdom and wonderful stories. Respectful listening can encourage the older person to share a wealth of experience and can result in a rewarding communication.

Responding to Older Persons

Verbal Skills

In the two-way process of communication, there is a sharing of ideas, knowledge, thoughts, and feelings. Each person listens, speaks, observes,

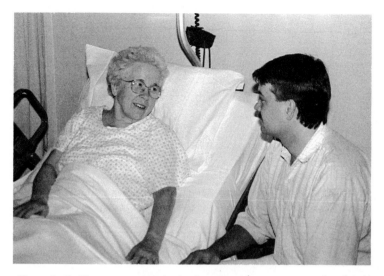

Figure 4–2. Two-way communication is easier with eye contact, a relaxed, calm position, empathy, and respect.

and feels from a personal frame of reference and frame of mind (Fig. 4–2). Choice of words and even their meaning are influenced by a person's unique situation especially in states of stress or anxiety.

Word exchange is not necessarily communication and a meeting of the minds. It is common in this society to say one thing and mean another, or ask one question and want an answer to another. "Beating around the bush" has become habitual for many people. The attempt to convey meaning in speech requires one to use verbal skills. A verbal skill is the ability to use words in a precise way in order to respond to and to develop communication. In any setting, the nurse is continually seeking or giving information and moral support. None of this is possible without verbal skills that clarify and expand on the nurse's understanding of the *person* with whom she is interacting.

Reflective Response

To reflect is to give back a likeness. In a "reflective response," one accurately repeats the gist of the message that has been received, by paraphrasing, or restating the message. Remember that a message may have three components: words, thoughts, and feelings. By responding to *all* that is offered by the speaker, the nurse shows that she is listening and not just repeating words. On the other hand, to avoid making a judgement, the nurse must be careful that she responds *only* to what has been offered. Restatement of simple comments can be helpful:

Patient: "I don't want breakfast."
Nurse: "You don't want breakfast."

If used too often, however, this technique of reflection will sound like an echo. In giving nursing care, reflective listening and paraphrasing can reduce generalizations to specific complaints and open the way for problem solving. Here is an example:

Patient: "Nobody gives me fresh water!"
Nurse: "You sound unhappy because you don't get fresh water."
Patient: "I don't have any *now*."

Communication flows when there is trust, and we tend to trust those who listen to us.

Clarification

A "clarification response" acknowledges a message and elaborates on it, asking the patient for verification, as in this example:

Patient: "Every time I want to talk to that doctor he is in and out of here so fast it hardly pays to open my mouth."
Nurse: "I think you're saying you want to talk to your doctor and you haven't had the chance."

In elaborating the nurse must be careful not to add any new information. If the nurse had said, "It sounds like he does that a lot," she would have been adding information. Although her assumption might have been correct, there is a good chance it might have been incorrect. Besides, this information would probably lead to a discussion about the doctor rather than the patient's real concern.

Certain phrases introduce a clarifying statement:

"Do I understand that . . . "
"I think you are saying . . . "
"Let's see if I am hearing you . . . "

Such clarifying statements prompt the person to whom they are said to go on and clarify even more. In instances where a long message has been given, summarizing can be an effective means of clarification.

The Use and Misuse of Questions

Questions are open or closed. "Open questions" begin with "how" and "what." They generally encourage communication because they ask for an explanation or description:

"How can I make you more comfortable?"
"What kinds of activity make your back hurt?"

Asking open questions of older persons, especially if they are ill, means patiently waiting for answers while they process and return information. This is an important way of allowing them to maintain control over what is happening.

Questions beginning with "when," "where," "which," and "who" are appropriate if the nurse is asking for specific information or a definite yes or no. The misuse of questions may occur in the act of making decisions for elderly persons. When acting in what one considers their "best interest," it is common to resort to this kind of questioning:

"Is it all right if . . . "
"Wouldn't you rather . . . "
"Don't you think it would be a good idea if . . . "
"How about if . . . "
"Shall I" . . . "Will you" . . . and so on.

Although it may *seem* polite or helpful to ask questions in this manner, it is condescending and should not be done. "Why" questions are open-ended in that they encourage explanations and request facts. However, they seek justification and put the person who is obliged to give it on the defensive. In interactions with older persons, this is disastrous, so avoid these kinds of questions:

"Why are you wearing two sweaters?"
"Why are you taking two blood pressure pills?"
"Why don't you want to eat breakfast?"

These questions imply that the older person to whom they are addressed is confused or childish, even though the intention may simply be to get helpful information.

Nonverbal Communication

In relating to others, words are combined with actions, expressions, and feelings. The body, mind, and soul cannot be separated in the communication process. We communicate even when we are totally silent. Nonverbal means of communication operate along with the verbal, but the speaker often is not conscious of this. Verbal and nonverbal behaviors can give conflicting messages. Nonverbal communication is described as "body language." For discussion purposes, nonverbal methods of communication will be classified as follows:

Expressions and movements
Postures
Behavior patterns that are routine, rituals
Use of objects

Expressions and Movements

Facial expressions and head, hand, and arm movements are a sort of sign language that enlarge or emphasize words and punctuation. "Affect" is a facial expression that displays a mood or emotion in a culturally defined way. In other words, an affect is how we are *supposed to look* based on how we feel. Affect can be inappropriate. For example, the nurse tells an older patient that it is "all right" that he spilled a glass of water. A frown on her face would deny her words, as would a smile on her lips but not in her eyes.

Older persons often search for signs of understanding and approval in a nurse's face when they are anxious and fearful. In circumstances under which speech is difficult and hearing is poor, the facial expression of the nurse an older person is communicating with may be the only way he can identify acceptance or rejection.

Widened eyes and the head tilted forward and a little to one side can be a sign that the nurse is paying attention. Raising the eyebrows alerts the older listener to a question. Smiling, nodding, shaking the head, and using hand movements for emphasis may work when words are not enough. Giving directions or descriptions to older persons is simplified when the hands do some of the communicating, although pointing should be avoided.

Normal movements that are necessary to everyday life speak a language in the way they are performed. For example, a nurse who is conducting a blood pressure clinic at a senior citizens apartment complex may reveal by the manner in which she sets up equipment whether she is glad to be there or is in a hurry to be gone.

Postures

The way in which one sits or stands communicates mood or attitude. Posture is an excellent way of demonstrating respect and interest in what the speaker is saying. These are some rules to follow:

- Avoid crossing your arms and legs. Such positions are associated with a closed mind.
- An open mind is suggested when you stand or sit with knees and feet slightly apart and hands and arms not touching the body.

- Maintain eye contact and lean slightly forward.
- Assume a position similar to that of the other person whenever possible.
- Remember that *comfort* influences posture. For example, crossing the arms and legs may indicate a person is "chilly." A chair may be uncomfortable and affect the manner in which one sits. This is one way in which environment influences communication.

The significance of posture is frequently lost on the very old person, who has all he can do to relate to details, without translating body language. Nevertheless, the nurse should remain aware of *her* posture in all interactions.

Behavior Patterns

An awareness of the routines and rituals that order our lives can play a major role in successful communication with aging people. The *ways* in which we offer apology, greeting, or sympathy, for instance, contribute to the verbal message. Our behaviors are established for social rituals, such as birthdays, weddings, and funerals. Personal routines also involve established behavior. Nursing care plans for older patients must take into account the personal routines of the individual, both to promote communication and to meet needs. The nurse who demonstrates caring by adhering to her older patient's bedtime routine is communicating very effectively. This patient will respond to the nurse when information is needed because the nurse has treated him or her with understanding and respect.

Use of Objects

"Keeping up with the Joneses" is one way of communicating with peers. However, material possessions also tell a story of pride, love, regard for beauty or utility, and the extent of intellectual curiosity. In home health nursing, this mode of communication helps fill in the background of the patient and family, paving the way for more interaction. For example, a large piano in the living room or an abundance of house plants offers information about someone with whom the nurse is communicating.

One's possessions are a display of one's values (Fig. 4-3). The elderly patient is telling the nurse this by asking that personal belongings, such as a photograph and clock, be close to the bedside. Self-esteem is communicated by a makeup kit. These are not simply quirks or ingrained habits, but part of a dynamic personality in communication with the surrounding world.

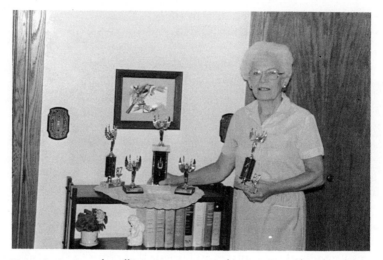

Figure 4–3. A trophy collection communicates this woman's pride in her ability to excel as a ballroom dancer at age 83.

The Importance of Touch

Touch is the means by which human beings begin to learn about their world when they are infants. To a great extent, words replace touch as one grows older. Occasions for touching are defined by society and are more explicitly defined within family and peer groups. Touch is generally acceptable only among close relatives, friends, and significant others. Touching, hugging, and holding are separate from sexual desire, yet they are often misinterpreted, so touch as a sign of understanding and acceptance should be used with care by the nurse (Fig. 4–4). Persons for whom touch has become a spontaneous gesture may be embarrassed when others misunderstand and become rigid or pull away when touched. Thus, instead of being a positive means of communication, touch can be a block. But to be deprived of touch is to be cold and lonely and is perhaps the cruelest form of rejection.

Older persons—and the older they are the more this is true—may remain untouched because they have lost those to whom they were closest. They *need* to be touched or at least given the opportunity to accept or reject closeness. Some people are reluctant to touch the skin of an older person because of its wrinkles, sclerotic or spidery blood vessels, uneven color, and dryness. Denial of the aging process is responsible for this negative reaction.

The nurse communicates caring by touching older patients with gentleness and acceptance. This is affective touch. Touch can reduce anxiety.

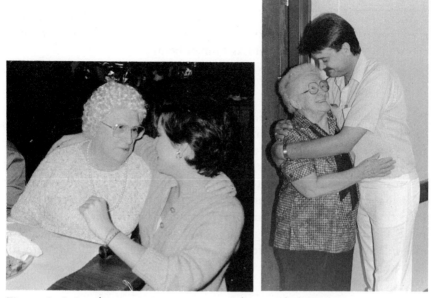

Figure 4–4. In the appropriate context, touching and hugging can communicate understanding.

Holding the hand of an aging patient when explaining procedures or asking questions promotes cooperation, inspires trust, and improves communication. Even task-oriented touch such as taking a pulse can communicate caring when touch is gentle and the nurse's manner is warm.

Learning from Older Persons

Communicating with Older Relatives

A look at relationships with older persons who are family members, friends, or simply acquaintances is a starting point for the nurse in learning to communicate with older persons. The insight gained from examining these interactions will also help the nurse grow as a person who, herself, is aging. One hopes that this will result in a deeper commitment to advocacy for the aging population. For example, the nurse who can identify whether or not she talks at, instead of to, her older relatives will be sensitive to this possibility in her work and will learn to avoid it.

When we talk *at* older persons because it takes too much time to talk *to* them, we devalue their years of accumulated wisdom. Failure to include them in the problem-solving aspects of family life because it takes too much effort devalues them as human beings.

Role Expectations

Role expectations of older persons inhibit communication by preventing one from seeing the individual and his specific needs. A classic example is the behavior expected from a parent. A parent is supposed to behave like a parent and take charge of his or her life, no matter what happens. If, as parents grow older, they fail to do this, they are often expected to submit to being treated like children by children who are now parents or of parenting age. Making decisions for and about older relatives often is more convenient than making an objective assessment. The results can be misunderstandings, injured feelings, missed messages, and a failure to communicate.

CASE STUDY

An 80-year-old father becomes unable to do the kind of repairing and building he has done all his life, and his family feels he should sit down and "take it easy." Since relaxing is something he has always had difficulty doing, he cannot stop working now. Has his personality changed? Has he become hard to handle because he is restless?

CASE STUDY

A 30-year-old man says the following: "You'd think with my mother dead two years, my Dad could learn to entertain himself or find somebody? No sir! He comes over here and he's like one of the kids. I hate to get on his back any more than I do. When I even mention it, he tells me he knows he's a bother and should be in a nursing home. But there are all kinds of widows where he lives. Will he ask one of them out? Not him! He'd rather feel sorry for himself."

The father in question here was dependent on his wife for social direction and "mothering" for almost 40 years. With that wife gone, he cannot function, at least at this point. The son expects him either to become independent enough to entertain himself or to find another woman to become dependent upon. Since he has failed to live up to his son's expectations, the father is labeled as a case of self-pity, when, given his personality and past relationship, his actions and reactions are normal.

Observing Body Language

Older men do not often cry. How do they communicate the feelings that should bring tears? One nurse learned this from observing her father:

> I never saw my Dad cry, but he had a habit of dropping his lower jaw and shifting it sideways when it seemed like everyone else was crying. It was real obvious, but maybe that was because I saw him do it all my life. After I thought about this a while, I began to notice that many of my older male patients shift their jaws or faces around when they are hurting.

How do the older people we know *look* when sad, fearful, happy, or contented? Can we learn anything about the body language of older people, in general, from our observations? Here is another nurse's story:

> Whenever I hear or read about crossed legs and arms meaning the person is closed or not listening, I get this picture in my mind of Uncle Charlie, who died when I was a teenager. But I used to go visit him when I was little. I will never forget how he looked sitting with his cronies on the bench outside the bank. He would sit for hours with his arms folded and legs folded and a pipe in his mouth. If he was being closed, it was a comfortable, relaxed, closing that I think meant he was content to be by himself, *inside* himself. I wonder now, when older patients sit like that, if it's not because they're being the same way, and those times are not good times to talk to them. Maybe they are okay alone?

Communication Barriers Due to Age

By growing old, a person becomes a treasure trove of history, humor, and wisdom, all of which should be shared. Yet, because of what aging involves, there are some natural barriers to successful sharing.

Passage of Time

The perception of time is a dimension that is affected by age. Years seem to pass more quickly as one grows older. This is true, even when a day "drags by." Think about when you first said, "I can't believe it's winter already," or when your birthday suddenly came too soon (see "How Long is a Long Time?").

The difference in perception of time means that years and incidents run together when one attempts to pinpoint definite dates along with

How Long is a Long Time?

A 52-year-old woman tells this story:

> A beautiful little girl gave me two weatherbeaten but fragrant lilacs. It was an impulse, I know. She ran across the street toward me, green backpack and long silky, brown hair flying in the breeze.
>
> "Here!" she said, and thrust the lilacs at me, blue eyes and freckles sparkling.
>
> "Why, thank you. They're beautiful. Where did you get them?" She pointed. "Off them ly-lee bushes."
>
> We crossed the street together. "Are you through with school for the day?" I asked.
>
> She hopped up the curb and nodded. "Yes! And I'm going to be in first grade next year."
>
> "Will you like that?"
>
> She hesitated a few seconds, but only to find the right words. Then, with a little jump, she exclaimed, "Ye-es, I've been in kintygarten eight years!"
>
> I smiled and thought about that as I went on my way. I'm sure I once felt that way myself. And now, it seems, I get a new phone book every two weeks!"

events. Conversation with an older person can be frustrating because of this, and the nurse can mistakenly label that person as disoriented, confused, or suffering long-term memory loss. This highlights the importance of careful listening and reflective response.

The Problem in Seeing Eye to Eye

Just as younger adults are guilty of talking at older adults instead of to them, older persons on occasion will totally ignore those younger than themselves. A camaraderie that stems from a common history and that younger people cannot share makes this natural. A young woman, for example, trying to do volunteer work with older women in a church social center, may be intimidated and feel inadequate when excluded from their conversation.

She may become resentful and may conclude that these women think "they know more than she does" — and they do! Most likely that's what is really bothering her. The older women may or may not be conscious of what they are doing. The point is that seeing eye to eye across a span of years can be impossible unless an effort is made to share experiences and ideas.

Short-term Memory Deficit

Short-term memory deficits are normal in the aged. The older person often has a clearer idea of what happened 20 years ago than he does of what happened last week. He may not recall what he said, and this forces him to be repetitive. However, the elderly person who constantly tells the same story or asks the same question ought to be closely listened to for whatever else he or she might be trying to say.

In the hospital, the older patient who asks the same question or relates the same incident more than once may or may not have short-term memory loss. Besides giving the appropriate response, the nurse must determine if that patient has the following needs:

- Needs clarification of what happened ("I had to go to X-ray three times today for the same thing.")
- Has a problem believing or understanding an explanation of a condition or treatment ("How long before my arm is healed?")
- Needs to discuss a concern and verbalize feelings ("My doctor told me I'd be walking good as new in a month. How can that be?")

The Effect of Sensory Losses

Decreased visual acuity and a gradual loss of hearing are signs of advancing age. A lot of middle-aged and older persons would rather squint than wear glasses. To many people, hearing aids are unacceptable.

The progressive hearing loss associated with a high percentage of the elderly population is an obstacle to satisfactory interaction with others. The concentration required to listen when one cannot hear well is tiring, so an older person listens selectively. The old saying, "He hears what he wants to hear," has basis in fact.

Hearing aids are considered by many to be a nuisance because they take time to become accustomed to, adjustment can be tricky, and sound may be distorted. Too often, the would-be wearers turn them off or never put them on. The nurse should be familiar with hearing aids and how they operate. She should be able to change batteries and insert ear molds. Positive reinforcement that the device is helpful to the nurse as well as the patient is necessary: "Mrs. S, I know about hearing aids, but they're not all exactly the same. Tell me how I sound to you and what I should do so you can hear me."

To lose one's hearing means social isolation. A vision loss cuts one off from things, but a hearing loss separates one from people. A lot of effort is required to communicate with someone who has impaired hearing. When several persons are interacting, it is tempting to exclude the older person who is hard of hearing. This may make him feel as if the others are talking about him. Older persons who do not hear well may be labeled uncooperative, belligerent, and senile.

It is always appropriate for the nurse to question an elderly person about the quality of his hearing at the beginning of a conversation: "Mr. K, please tell me if my voice bothers you, if I am speaking too loud, or if you cannot hear me."

When an older person indicates that a hearing problem is present, it is also appropriate to ask if one ear is better than the other and then speak more closely to that ear.

In an unfamiliar environment, a comfort level must be established before communication can begin. Reducing all stimuli will be helpful. Elderly persons may not be able to tune out distracting noises, so radios and televisions should automatically be turned off. With or without a hearing aid, the older listener needs time to process what has been heard and then give an answer.

When communicating with the hearing-impaired older person, observe the following guidelines:

- Address the person by name to attract his attention.
- Face him and be sure he can see your face.
- Speak slowly and clearly, and do not shout or exaggerate your lip movements (Fig. 4–5). Elderly people who are hard of hearing

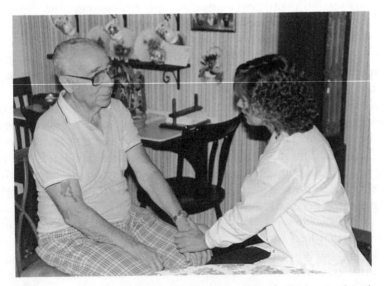

Figure 4–5. Face the hearing-impaired person and speak clearly. Touch and posture help communicate caring and acceptance.

learn to do some lipreading, which is difficult because many sounds "look alike."

- Use facial expressions, gestures, and body language along with your words.
- Speak in short sentences or phrases and allow time between them for response.
- When the person does not understand what you've said, rephrase your message using different words. Be careful not to raise your voice when doing this.

Hearing loss is not restricted to very old people. It is not uncommon for the middle-aged to begin to experience this problem, and they can be extremely sensitive about it. The nurse must be alert to facial expressions, such as a frown or look of intense concentration, and the slight turning of the head that may signal better hearing in one ear.

Hearing is easier when one can see what is happening, but visual overload should be avoided. During a new experience, an older person may become alarmed if there are too many things happening at the same time, like a number of people moving around — even if that movement is normal, such as in a hospital room. If another patient is being brought on a stretcher to the bed next to the older patient, it is not a good time for the nurse to talk about planned routines.

Poor vision can be a barrier to communication. The older person should have his glasses on during interactions, and the lighting should be sufficient so he can see the speaker's face. A tendency to raise one's voice when addressing older patients with poor vision who wear thick eyeglasses is common. The nurse must be careful not to do this, because sensory losses do not necessarily go together. When the patient does not see well, the nurse must rely entirely on verbal skills and touch to convey a message.

Confusion and disorientation in the elderly may prevent communication altogether. These conditions may be temporary and related to the present environment, overstimulation, or a hearing loss.

Vocal Cues and Silence

How one says what one says, or says nothing at all, are components of the communication process. Sarcasm or affection can be sent in the same word just as interest or disinterest, concern or annoyance can be communicated in the same phrase.

"Wonderful!" can mean wonderful, or not wonderful at all, depending on the voice. In like manner, "Let me help you," can sound insincere.

Vocal cues penetrate barriers when words do not. The emphasis placed on words, the pitch and volume of speech, may be all that is heard when someone is under stress. Consider this common exchange:

Doctor: "What did the nurse tell you yesterday?"
Patient: "I don't know, but she sounded in a hurry."

It is important to learn how and when to remain silent and to understand what silence means to the older person. When the nurse is silent while caring for an older patient it may be misconstrued as rejection, especially if that patient cannot see well or is hard of hearing. Silence can only be comfortable when that comfort is mutual. One way to assure that it will be is to tell the patient that you are listening for anything he needs to ask or say while you work. When the nurse becomes engrossed in the task at hand and unable to talk she should explain what is happening: "I'm going to concentrate on this I.V., Mrs. K, but I'm listening."

During the busy hospital day, when people are in and out all the time, the older patient may feel the need for some peace and quiet and react to this need by closing his eyes and becoming quiet himself. The nurse must be aware that this is not a sign of depression. In the middle of the night when unable to sleep, the older person may react to the silence by wanting another person to share it. At either of these times, holding the patient's hand for a few minutes communicates understanding.

Space

The distance that should be maintained between two people who are communicating is an important factor in establishing effective communication (Fig. 4 – 6). Space needs vary depending on culture, background, feelings, and personality.

Consider how some people come close to you during conversations and how others tend to step back once an initial greeting is exchanged. Loss of hearing and poor eyesight place older people at a disadvantage. Elderly patients will usually allow the nurse to come close enough to touch them as she talks. Still, she must be alert for signs of discomfort, pulling away, hunching shoulders, turning the head, or averting or closing the eyes. The immobile elderly are particularly vulnerable, so they must be approached with great gentleness.

General Blocks to Communication

The nurse can block communication with the older person in the following ways:

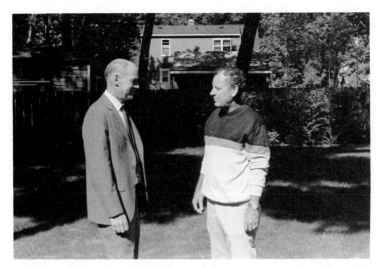

Figure 4–6. The right amount of space makes communication easier and more effective.

Improper questioning
Inappropriate reassurance
Giving advice/making judgements
Praising or scolding
Yes or no answers
Defending
Anger, or misunderstanding its use

Improper Questioning

When using questions, avoid asking "why" and calling for yes or no responses unless absolutely indicated. Asking appropriate questions means listening for answers and refraining from interjecting what one supposes to be the forthcoming reply. Remember it takes more time for older persons to process what they hear, to organize thoughts, and to formulate an answer.

Inappropriate Reassurance

The best of intentions go into giving some of the most ineffective reassuring responses. Many of them are cliches:

"Perhaps it is the Lord's will."
"Things could be worse."
"There, there."

Statements beginning with "At least it's not . . . " or "Be thankful that . . . " are just as bad. On the face of it, these types of reassurance might seem comforting, but they are not. At the very least, they suggest to the person to whom they are directed that he should resign himself to his fate. If the concern under discussion is creating a lot of anxiety, this suggestion may make the anxious person resentful, frustrated, and angry. It is important to remember that the magnitude of problems and concerns is different for each person. The age difference between nurse and patient may make understanding more difficult. Going to the supermarket may be an irksome task for a young nurse with a full-time job and a new baby, but it may be the only time all week the older person gets out of her apartment; to be deprived of this event by a health problem can be disastrous to morale.

Giving Advice/Making Judgments

Even when advice appears to be sorely needed, it should not be given. In problem solving, "If I were you . . . " or "If you want my opinion . . . " are clearly the wrong way to press a point, however worthy it may be. Statements of "ought to" and "should" or "should not" also fall into the category of giving advice or making judgments.

To suggest is proper and is not the same as giving advice. Distinguishing between the two can be a matter of words instead of ideas — how you say what you say:

"You ought to get out of bed at 11 o'clock and then you'd feel like staying up for lunch." Although "You eat better sitting in a chair," may be the idea, the better way to express it is, "Think about getting out of bed just before lunch, and see if you are more comfortable eating when you can sit in a chair."

An older person, like everyone else, should be part of his own decision-making process whenever possible. In the ill elderly, dependency is reinforced when the nurse offers advice or makes judgments, even though this hastens problem solving and seems to be in the patient's "best interests." Advice and judgments stem from personal opinions and values and discourage the patient from expressing his or her own opinions.

Praising or Scolding

Recognition of what the person has achieved or is trying to do is preferable to giving praise, as praise can be intimidating. To say, "You did a wonderful job of giving your own insulin," may leave the new diabetic afraid to ask a question. "You followed the right steps in giving yourself insulin," said with a smile, would be more effective communication.

Scolding, even in a jolly manner, "What am I going to do with you, you didn't swallow your pills again?" is demeaning and may accomplish nothing except to reinforce the negative behavior. A statement of what happened, "You didn't swallow your pills," may or may not prompt an explanation but is the best reaction.

Yes or No Answers

Just as the nurse must refrain from asking yes or no questions, she should not give yes or no answers when an opinion is requested. An older person seeking agreement with feelings or behavior should be encouraged to express his or her values and choices. Sometimes this results in a going-in-circles sort of interaction, yet it is revealing and may help identify an anxiety or a problem.

In the following example, an elderly resident of an apartment complex talks to a nurse who has come to teach a class on cardiac rehabilitation:

Resident: "I have such pain in these shoulders, it's hard to move this old walker. Is Tylenol any good for that?"
Nurse: "You sound as if you think it might be."
Resident: "I just wondered."
Nurse: "For some people it is very good; so is aspirin."
Resident: "My doctor says not to take aspirin. Bad for my stomach. I don't know."
Nurse: "What does he say about this pain you are having?"
Resident: "He doesn't say anything."
Nurse: "You might try some plain or extra-strength Tylenol."
Resident: "I got some pain pills from the doctor."
Nurse: "If you show me what they are, I can be more helpful."

She goes and gets her bottle of prescription pills, which are Tylenol with codeine.

Nurse: "What did he say these were for?"
Resident: "Same thing."
Nurse: "They're for the pain in your shoulders?"
Resident: "They don't help."
Nurse: "Maybe when you talk to your doctor again, you can talk that over with him."
Resident: "He'll just tell me I'm getting arthritis again. That's all he ever says."

Nurse: "Tell me what you know about arthritis."
Resident: "Nothing. I'll get crippled up like Selma."

Fears and concerns have now been identified, and the nurse can be helpful to this woman by educating her on the facts of arthritis.

Defending

Complaints about care and criticisms of care-givers in the hospital or nursing home are handled quickly, but ineffectively, when the nurse assumes the role of defender. Because she is in a position of authority the nurse can explain or make excuses, whichever seems appropriate. However, both options close the door on any meaningful communication with the patient, as his feelings are ignored and the possibility of a problem is denied. This is an example:

Patient: "I can't stand that night nurse, she hurries me when I have to go
　　　　to the bathroom. I can't *go* fast. I'll fall."
Nurse: "Perhaps you called her at a busy time, and anyway, as long as
　　　　she's with you, you can't fall."

This will be the end of the conversation. The nurse has defended the action of a peer and the patient is left to deal with anxiety and fear alone.

The use of reflective response is probably a good beginning in getting to the heart of the problem: "You are afraid you will fall at night."

Anger or Misunderstanding Its Use

Anger is a major block to communication, and it depletes energy that could be spent in building a positive interpersonal relationship. An angry person provokes anger in others. Anger in a sick older person can be a means of expressing frustration and anxiety due to loss of control and to unmet needs. In the nurse, anger may be a reaction to what she perceives as a failure of the patient to cooperate and respond to nursing actions.

Even when it is short-lived, anger can spread and create a rippling effect far from where it originated. The patient becomes angry when the nurse suggests he feed himself, and he complains to his physician. The physician becomes angry and writes an order to feed the patient at his request. The nurse becomes angry at the physician and when X-ray calls to request that another patient be brought down to that department, the nurse is angry on the phone. The receptionist at the radiology desk snaps at her coworker, and so on. All of this occurs because there is a lack of understanding about what caused the original *symptom* of anger. Anger is a symptom, and understanding the cause is essential to effective communication. In this example, the nurse could go back to the patient and ask, "What can I do to make it easier for you to feed yourself?"

Communicating with the Confused Elderly Patient

An elderly patient who enters the hospital may be temporarily disconnected from reality by the shock of sudden illness or injury. When that person attempts to reconnect, the result may be panic and helplessness at finding himself in an unfamiliar world. In one way or another, this person asks for help or tries to help himself. He cries out, bangs on the bedrail, or tries to get out of bed. The nurse evaluates this patient as being confused, which he is. Yet a simple contact with another human being may be all he needs to come back to the present.

Confusion is increased if the nurse communicates alarm by her tone of voice and her actions. The patient may become agitated and unmanageable and may agitate the nurse. A relaxed approach to this kind of situation is difficult, yet may be the only one that is workable. The nurse should speak in a soft, low voice, identifying herself and making simple, reassuring statements such as, "You are safe." Perhaps she can ask, "Tell me what's wrong."

Holding the patient's hand may help him to feel safe and permit some organization of his thoughts. When the patient does not fully comprehend what is happening, he will depend on the nurse's facial expression, touch, and tone of voice to guide him to a place where he is comfortable. Frequently, all that the confused elderly patient needs is extra time and patience or, truly, some "TLC." A perfect example of this is also a familiar one. The nursing student, who typically has more time to spend with patients, finishes bathing her elderly patient, assists her into a chair, and then sits with her the rest of the morning, smiling, listening, and asking questions. Her report to the instructor is prefaced by "The nurse told me Mrs. R is confused at times. I didn't think she was confused at all."

Family members are often embarrassed and distressed by confusion in their elderly relative, especially if that person was not previously confused. Comfort should be offered by the nurse. The family may need hugs and verbal support so that they can interact with their loved one in a satisfactory way. They need to know their mother or father is experiencing a state that is common and almost predictable in the elderly hospitalized patient. Methods of communicating that have worked for the nurse, such as touching and reassuring, will be beneficial to the family.

The Nurse as an Interviewer

An interview is the giving or sharing of data in a purposeful way to reach a goal. Questions are asked and answers given to expand on what is known about a particular subject. In nursing, the interview is a part of assessment (see Chap. 2) and has the following four goals:

- To identify and clarify health needs and goals
- To provide a way for an individual to express feelings
- To instruct
- To offer support

The nurse systematically directs the person being interviewed through the process of explaining and discussing the available information. The success of the interview depends on how well the nurse and the individuals involved are able to communicate with one another.

Working with older persons offers the nurse many opportunities to assume the role of interviewer. The kind and amount of data that must be obtained, shared, and processed will vary according to the setting and individual situation. Nurses and older people interact in health promotion or wellness programs, in medical clinics, independent practice, the home, hospitals, and extended care institutions like nursing homes.

A physically and emotionally comfortable climate must be established for a successful interview. When external stimuli such as temperature, light, sound, and odors are beyond her control, the nurse should recognize that they can affect communication. In the patient's home, where he is in control, the nurse might have to adjust to distractions that are part of the patient's normal existence. He can probably pet the frisky dog jumping up between him and the nurse and answer questions at the same time, while the nurse may be unable to concentrate.

Planning enough time for the interview and remaining flexible are key factors. An interview, no matter where the information is eventually used, is always conducted as a matter of privacy and confidentiality. The first step in the actual interview process is for the nurse to introduce herself, if this is her first interaction with the older person, or if some time has elapsed since the last interview.

When the nurse does not know the older person, she must note his mental acuity early in the interview. The accuracy and credibility of the information being given can then be determined. Generally speaking, the older the person is, the more important it is to give him time to talk about himself and the purpose of the interview. This will shed some light on his mental faculties and on the language level the nurse should use when speaking.

In ongoing assessment, when the patient obviously recognizes the nurse, it is appropriate to say, without an introduction, "Mr. C, the last time we talked about this we . . . " and reiterate and review.

It is never a good idea for the nurse to begin an interview with an older person by asking, "Do you remember me?" Short-term memory loss is aggravating to the older adult, and any reminder that it exists is unwelcome. All verbal and nonverbal skills are incorporated into the act of interviewing.

Rewarding Communication

If the nurse makes each contact with the older person a sincere effort to listen and understand, communication will naturally follow. When in doubt as to how to begin, the nurse should relate on a personal, human level. The results can be amazing:

> None of us really enjoyed taking care of Clara. She was bitter about losing her leg and depressed about losing her husband, all understandable, of course, but hard to deal with because she never talked to anybody. At 70, which isn't that old any more, she seemed ready to give up.
>
> Then one morning I went in her room and opened the blinds, and the day was enough to depress *anyone*. I said, "Why is it always grayer in November?"
>
> And Clara answered, "November woods are bare and brown, November woods are still."
>
> I was so surprised! I asked her if it was from a poem and she said, "I don't know." But then I asked her some more about poetry (I love it!) and found out she had read a lot of poetry to her classes when she taught sixth grade. I was so glad to have found something to get her to talk about.

The sharing of simple thoughts and observations often invites response from the older person with whom one is trying to communicate, which can be a first step in building a positive interpersonal relationship.

Summary

Communication is a two-way process that demands skill both in listening and responding. Proper listening shows respect and empathy for the speaker. Verbal skills include knowing how to respond in order to keep communication flowing. Asking questions that require more than yes and no answers is important. Nonverbal communication is body language, the use of gestures, objects, and touch. Knowing when to be silent enhances communication.

The nurse can learn about communication barriers due to age by observing her own relationships with older persons. Role expectations, perception of time, inability to share experiences, and sensory deficits affect how we communicate. General communication blocks are the use of improper response, defensiveness, and anger. Communicating with the confused elderly patient is less frustrating if the nurse learns to recognize the cause of confusion. In interviewing older persons, the nurse uses verbal and nonverbal skills, allows ample time for the interview, and considers what effect the environment could have on the outcome.

Activities

1. Think about the conversations you have with older relatives. When might you find these persons boring? When might you find them interesting?
2. Make a list of six general points to remember when you are about to ask for information from a hospitalized older person.
3. Read the following, write three possible responses that you could give. Identify which verbal skills you are using.

   Mrs. R is 86 years old and was admitted to the hospital four days ago with a heart condition. She is mentally alert. At 6 P.M. you answer her call light and she says: "Nurse, I have to go home. I want to go home. My daughter can take care of me."

4. In conversations with three different persons of any age, note the nonverbal communication that took place and what was being said at the time.
5. Discuss how your possessions can communicate your values.
6. Have a conversation (ten minutes) with another student, while your ears are plugged with cotton. Then reverse the situation. Discuss what you "heard" and your feelings.

Bibliography

Burgoon M, Ruffner M: Human Communication. New York, Holt, Rinehart & Winston, 1978

Ebersole P, Hess P: Toward Healthy Aging. Human Needs and Nursing Responses, 2nd ed. St. Louis, CV Mosby, 1985

Long L, Prophit Sr P: Understanding/Responding. Monterey, CA, Wadsworth, 1981

Montgomery C: What you can do for the confused elderly. Nursing 17:55–56, 1987

Sontora G: Communicating better with the elderly. Nurs Life 4:24–27, 1986

Tisdale S: The one patient I couldn't nurse. RN 51:34–35, 1988

Yurick A, Spier B, Robb S, et al: The Aged Person and the Nursing Process, 2nd ed. Norwalk, CT, Appleton Century Crofts, 1984

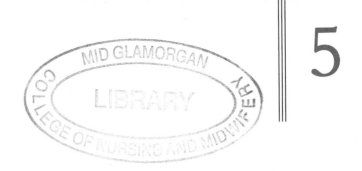

5

Psychosocial Adjustment to Aging

Learning Objectives

When you complete this chapter, you should be able to:

1. Define "psychosocial adjustment."
2. Identify the kinds of loss experienced in aging.
3. Discuss factors that make retirement a satisfying time of life.
4. Describe what an older person with high self-esteem might be like.
5. List roles that are possible for older persons.
6. Explain ways in which the nurse can identify and reduce stress in older patients.
7. Write three statements that could be made to an older patient to help maintain his self-esteem.

Individual differences make each older person interesting and unique. In the famous speech he delivered on his 70th birthday, Mark Twain said, "I have achieved my seventy years in the usual way: by sticking strictly to a scheme of life which would kill anybody else. . . . we can't reach old age by another man's road."

Psychosocial adjustment to aging is a lifelong growth process of learning from the past, living fully in the present, and preparing for the future. This process is affected by who and what one is as a personality within a social and economic environment. Common potential stressors are related to loss, and adjustment to loss is a major task. Loss requires change of lifestyle, role, relationships, and philosophy. Maintaining self-esteem, finding a reason for getting out of bed in the morning, and having a purpose for living are all crucial to good psychosocial adjustment. The nurse should understand what the potential stressors in aging are in order to do complete interviews and assessments and to understand older people as individuals. Reducing stress for the aging patient and promoting self-esteem are nursing responsibilities.

Potential Stressors in Aging

Early Personality Development in Coping with Loss

A stage of development is a step toward completeness. This completeness is called "ego integrity" in old age, or a sense of fulfillment. Some psychologists, in defining the stages of a lifespan in personality development, have stated or implied that there are certain tasks or challenges related to each stage (see Chap. 3). Achievement or failure affects progression from stage to stage, overall growth, and completeness. This helps account for the way a person adapts or copes at any given age. For example, the person who never learns to trust may develop a suspicious nature. The potential for stress in the adaptations and adjustments to old age is greater in one who does not have ego integrity, because he or she may feel life has been empty. This is a fundamental loss and it will influence the way one handles other losses.

Loss in General

Loss is a part of living, and the longer one lives the more one loses. This is not to say there are no gains. But given the kinds of losses older persons have to bear, gains may be hard to identify. In the face of loss, strong attitudes, emotions, and memories surface along with new feelings to comfort or plague the older adult and determine how an adjustment is made. Sometimes the result is despair. Loss can be a chain reaction forcing an older person into making major decisions, as one elderly lady said, " . . . before it was *time*."

Here is her story:

> We had to sell our house before it was *time*. We planned on staying there for at least a couple more years. Then my husband had prostate surgery along with cancer. When the nurse had to quit coming, I wanted to sell the house and move into town. My husband didn't. I was taking care of his catheter but I was afraid. What if he got sick and I couldn't take care of him way out there? We had no neighbors. Well, one of our sons finally convinced his dad. We no sooner moved into an apartment and he died. If I'd have known that was going to happen so soon I'd have stayed put. Maybe he wouldn't have died then either.

The road to psychosocial adjustment as a widow, for this older woman, had obstacles that often confront people in her circumstances. Besides the sorrow that accompanies loss of a spouse, she had guilt and regrets over what had seemed to be a logical decision at the time. Loss leads to change, which results in a positive or negative adjustment. On the one hand, it would seem that this should get easier as one ages, since loss is expected. On the other, a long life means well-established habits, patterns, and relationships, and an accumulation of experiences and feelings. This is where consideration of the individual personality is critical in understanding the process of adjustment.

Specific Losses

Personal Appearance/Sexual Image

The loss of youthfulness in the mirror, the inability to read without eyeglasses, and the aches and pains that come more often and stay longer may be the first obvious changes of aging to which one must adjust. Maintaining physical attractiveness and mobility in a way that is personally comfortable is of the utmost importance in healthy adaptation. After all, what constitutes beauty in old age, or any age, is a matter of preference. So old people who dye their hair, have plastic surgery or embark on periodic "health kicks" to look and feel better may be very happy with *where* they are and only seek to improve *what* they are.

Psychosocial adjustment to the obvious changes due to advancing age is partially influenced by the sexual image, or the perception of how one relates to others as a male or female. Stress becomes a factor when an older person believes that satisfactory intimate or even friendly relationships are based on physical appearance. Failure to accept oneself as an older person means maladjustment as a member of an age group and, perhaps, loss of support.

Health

One often hears people say, "I don't mind getting old, I guess, as long as I'm healthy," or "When you have your health you have everything." Many people dread the approach of old age because, undeniably, there is a higher incidence of chronic disease. The multiple potential problems of aging promote dependency and discomfort. Specifically, they keep people, for whom time is running out, from doing what they want to do with that time.This may be more stressful than pain. With dependency comes loss of control, which is frightening. Loss of "good" health by one's own standards is stressful when it interferes with a life-style.

CASE STUDY

Mr. K retired at 62 from his construction job because he had major chest surgery. He had at least one serious bout with influenza or a chest cold every winter thereafter. His habitual drinking and poor eating habits did not incapacitate him in any way, but he did suffer from a gastric ulcer by the time he was 70. He was a pleasant, easygoing man who would have told you he was in good health as long as he was able to walk two miles to the next town every day, weather permitting. Once there he would spend four to six hours playing cards and drinking beer with his old friends. At 71 he fell and fractured his hip. Although his recovery was rapid and uneventful, he was no longer able to walk to town. Once a week a neighbor would give him a ride there and back. He actually looked better and his ulcer was less troublesome as a result of this life-style change. He drank less and he ate better because he was afraid he would get weak and fall again. Still, he began to have periods of depression over his state of health, now considering himself "not well."

Loss of good health by another's standards is stressful when that other person is in a position to initiate action or influence decisions. Often family members will insist on monitoring an older relative's living habits and making changes when they feel the older person's health will not permit them to remain in control. There are situations in which this may be warranted. More often, well-meaning significant others give advice where it is not wanted and create stress for an older person who wishes to adjust to a change in health status in his own way. There are older persons being pressured into surrendering their independence because they "are not well enough to be alone," or just the opposite may be the case. An elderly person may want to go to a nursing home and a kind offspring will not permit it, preferring to provide some assistance because, "I don't want to see my mother in a nursing home."

Loss of health in old age, especially due to a chronic medical problem, is stressful when the person, such as a spouse, on whom one depended for help or moral support is gone. Finally, changes in health status may be more stressful for those who have enjoyed excellent health most of their lives.

Retirement

Retirement, as a considerable period of time in one's life, is a new phenomenon. In the past, if people lived long enough to retire, they didn't live long enough to create any kind of new lifestyle. Retirement is a new frontier and full of unknowns. Satisfactory adjustment to retirement depends on many factors. How one views the loss of a work-role identity is only part of it. Stress may be caused by the conditions under which one retires, that is, whether it was optional and whether health was an issue. How well one plans for retirement has considerable impact. Insufficient income in retirement is a tremendous stressor because it affects all areas of life. Housing, food, and transportation are always major expenses. Concern over health care costs in older age, particularly, can overshadow the joy of anticipating the life of a retiree.

As one grows older, the meaning of "home" usually undergoes some changes. For married couples with families, a home that becomes an empty nest may suddenly be too big. Retirement may necessitate change of residence from a financial standpoint. Loss of physical strength or mobility or loss of a spouse can contribute to a decision to sell a home and move into a smaller dwelling. Disposing of the treasures of a lifetime is compulsory in such moves and constitutes losing part of one's identity. Advancing age and declining health may force an individual to live with someone or eventually move to a nursing home. Any of these changes can be stressful.

The excitement and fun of the best of retirement life-styles is not without loss. Leaving old neighborhoods or migrating to another climate means loss of friends, familiar leisure activities, and social roles. Lack of flexibility in the face of these readjustments induces stress. A new perspective on old relationships may be in order when married couples find themselves with more time to spend together (Fig. 5–1).

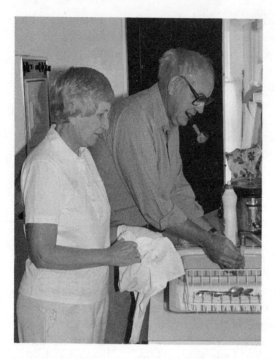

Figure 5–1. Retirement can mean growing with a spouse, sharing, and communicating in little ways.

Death of Others

When discussing aging and the deaths it brings, it is natural to focus on the loss of a spouse, siblings, and peers, probably in that order. Yet those who live to be very old frequently outlive their own children. Older people who come from large families or have large families of their own are likely to endure the heartbreaking loss of a young person. This kind of death in a family may be the hardest to bear and the grieving process can be endless.

One elderly woman whose 19-year-old only grandson was in a fatal automobile accident can no longer go to bed before 1:30 in the morning, the time she received the tragic news. An elderly man gets sick every year around Easter, which was when his 25-year-old daughter died of leukemia five years ago. The lasting pain of such memories affects many older people for the remainder of their lives. Outliving younger loved ones is not only traumatic, but it can elicit guilt feelings that persist for years: "Why didn't the Lord take me instead? She had her whole life ahead of her." This lament is familiar to anyone who knows an older person who has experienced this kind of loss.

Although many elderly people accept death as part of life, loss does not always get easier just because one gets older. An older woman may *say* after his death that her ailing husband is "peaceful now," or "better off," but her innermost feelings may be quite the opposite. The death of a spouse with whom one has lived for 50 years or more cannot be easy. Besides the sorrow it brings, such loss may mean significant changes in one's life. The loss of brothers, sisters, and peers adds to loneliness and heightens one's awareness that more loss, and one's own death, is imminent. This awareness is potentially stressful.

Divorce

Is one ever too old for a divorce? Apparently not. Although the divorce rate is not high in the 65+ age group, divorce must be considered as a potential stressor. The grief that accompanies this action is similar to that following the death of a spouse. Along with this grief comes a sense of failure.

Ethnic Factors

The term "ethnic" refers to a population or race of people classified according to shared customs and traits. Blacks, Hispanics, native American Indians, Alaskan natives, Japanese, and Chinese are examples of ethnic minority groups. Within each of these groups there are integrating beliefs, ideals, and traditional behaviors related to family, religion, and community. Historically, elderly people in all ethnic minorities were accorded respectful treatment. A couple of general statements can be made about these elderly people in today's society. Blacks, Hispanics, and native Americans have a higher incidence of chronic disease. Life expectancies for blacks and native Americans is shorter than for the others. Overall, the elderly in ethnic minority groups are poorer.

Remember that discrimination is associated with the definition of ethnic minority. Economic and educational development of these groups has been restricted. Racial prejudice and language are still barriers. Ethnic minorities tend not to use available health services because of pride, tradition, language problems, and often because they do not know such services exist. Where family bonds are not strong, the elderly may be in dire need. As younger generations of ethnic minorities assimilate the values and beliefs of others, their perspective on aging and the aged may well change. In turn, older family members, once revered and cared for, may not adapt positively to old age at all.

Poverty

A reliable estimate of the financial status of older people as a population cannot be obtained. There are too many regional discrepancies in the cost of services and goods and too many variables in the life of each individual. Although money cannot buy happiness, it does make psychosocial adjustment to old age more enjoyable and comfortable and health problems easier to manage. To be poor, and especially poor and old, creates a potential for stress (see Chap. 1).

Maintaining Self-Esteem

Definition of Self-Esteem for Old Age

Self-esteem means having confidence and satisfaction in self. In the context of old age, it means liking oneself well enough to keep going with dignity and self-acceptance to achieve inner peace and ego integrity. The older person with high self-esteem will be motivated to help others (Fig. 5–2). As one grows older, maintaining and developing self-esteem is the pinnacle of psychosocial adjustment.

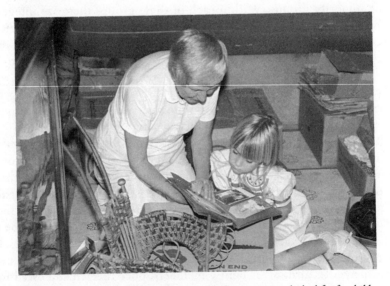

Figure 5–2. Self-esteem can motivate an older person to enrich the life of a child.

The Decision to Grow Older

There is a difference between *getting* older and *growing* older. Getting older is a grudging acceptance of what one cannot change and a reluctance to make decisions that will result in challenge, opportunity and, ultimately, personal satisfaction. For many people, for various reasons, this is the only way their old age can realistically happen. Unmet needs get in the way of an orderly and meaningful progression through old age. Role transitions that should be positive are incomplete and unrewarding. For example, when love and caring relationships have been lacking throughout life, an older person cannot be expected to change into a doting grandparent overnight. Role transitions that are naturally painful may be devastating, such as those of widowhood.

Independence is said to be one of the basic qualities that makes a person happy. Nevertheless, growing older has more possibilities when one realizes that some dependence often makes independence attainable. Here is an example:

A 90-year-old, unmarried woman lives alone. She dislikes having "strangers" in her house. Yet the regular services of a young woman who does her shopping and cleaning make it feasible for her to stay independent.

Interdependence can be mutually rewarding. Maggie Kuhn gave an excellent example in telling an audience that she could only reach out to others and share with them what she has learned if those others helped her as she climbed the steps to the podium.

There are those who insist they will go into old age kicking and screaming. A certain amount of kicking and screaming can be healthy if it is converted into positive energy and used to stay physically fit and useful. Universal law does not state that one has to like aging. On the other hand, it is a fact that in keeping an open mind and heart, one can learn to love aging. The secret then is to make aging *good*, by living and growing with it.

Those people who grow and develop into old age have chosen, consciously or unconsciously, between completing their identity or turning into poor old souls. They adapt to changing roles and recognize their usefulness to society. They have learned that not only is it permissible to change one's priorities but that in many cases it is also wise and quite comfortable. Personality traits may become more defined. Preferences and opinions surface in the process and influence the older person in making decisions. Even though this phenomenon may surprise or dismay others, to the older person it is part of self-discovery (Fig. 5–3). Main-

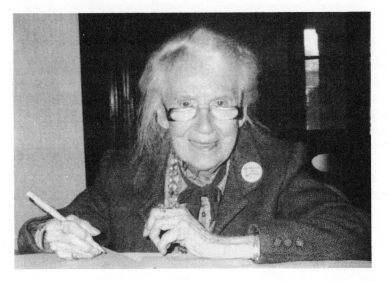

Figure 5 – 3. "The triumph over tragedies and failures, and disappointments and losses give you esteem and a certain self-confidence for the late years."—Maggie Kuhn

taining self-esteem involves accepting the years and one's own limitations and filling the roles that look promising.

About Roles

Roles are characterized by societal expectations with certain restraints and privileges that accompany function. One is born into family roles and expands those roles through emotional attachments and new relationships. For an older person, grandparenting is one such role. Work roles and social roles are achieved, some of which are more essential than others. One changes roles in an effort to meet continuing adult needs for caring relationships, some kind of recognition and influence, enjoyment, and independence.

Role transition frequently demands major adjustments of life-style, behavior patterns, and attitudes, and it may occur over a period of time with certain functions gradually being replaced by others. Crises occur when the change is sudden and there has been no preparation. Becoming a retiree can be one such crisis when a person has maintained an identity only through job or profession.

Preretirement Planning

Preretirement planning as a fringe benefit of employment is a valuable resource in positive socialization to old age. In many communities, local banks and investment firms offer programs for financial planning, a major component of preretirement planning on which all other aspects depend. When such services are unavailable, publications from the American Association of Retired Persons offer advice on numerous subjects.

Preretirement programs are generally structured for those over age 50. Topics for discussion and research include financial planning, Social Security benefits, supplemental health insurance, legal aspects such as wills, housing alternatives, myths and process of aging, nutrition, exercise, volunteerism, travel and hobbies, educational opportunities, and earning money in retirement. The company that plans such a program may choose to discuss its particular retirement options also. When a person has some choice as to the age he or she will retire, the transition from work role to that of retiree will be smoother.

The role of retiree encompasses many other roles (Fig. 5 – 4). Successful transition into a leisure role with no structured plan beyond utilizing community resources to enhance each day, live and learn, and make wise decisions is part of wellness (see Chap. 7).

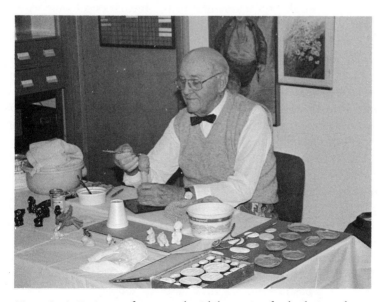

Figure 5 – 4. Retirement from a regular job leaves time for developing talents.

New Work Roles

No matter how inviting retirement appears, there are those people who just do not feel useful unless they are earning a paycheck. Furthermore, a reduced and fixed income may turn out to be insufficient for what the retired person needs or wants.

When making a living is not an issue, there are job opportunities at minimum wage for the retiree. The drop in the birth rate since 1964 means that the pool of youthful workers is drying up. For that reason many industries, particularly fast food chains, are targeting older people as prospective employees. The prevailing philosophy of such programs is that older workers are role models who have a stabilizing influence on the work force.

Volunteering

Volunteering is an excellent way for an older person to remain productive, to learn, and to feel needed. There is fierce competition for the services of volunteers in many communities, and the need seems to be growing. In health care alone, the list of tasks volunteers can learn to perform is endless. Transporting patients is one major area of need. Older persons function well as transport people in hospitals, as well as working, for instance, as Red Cross bus drivers. The concept of older people helping older people is instrumental in the formation of support groups and programs for counseling.

Two national and federally funded groups specifically for older people are the Foster Grandparent Program and Retired Seniors Volunteer Program, or R.S.V.P. Foster Grandparents need to be at least 60 years old. They make about two dollars an hour for 20 hours a week. Eligibility for entrance into this program, since it is paid, is based on income. Foster grandparents work in institutions, school districts, day care centers, and private homes to help children who have special needs. R.S.V.P. is also for seniors 60 or older. It offers its members various opportunities to contribute their time, knowledge, and experience to help others in the community. The program may operate a bit differently in different communities and serves as a clearinghouse for placing volunteers.

SCORE is the Service Corps of Retired Executives and is sponsored by the Small Business Administration. It requires that its volunteers have leadership ability and experience in some aspect of management. Their role is to advise small businesses. With about 13,000 volunteers in its ranks, SCORE has become nationwide in its scope.

The struggle some retirees have in coming to the conclusion that voluntcering is worthwhile busincss involvcs a shift in perspective: recognition of the fact that worth is not related to wealth. An example is Mr. S, who was anxious and restless upon retirement from a job where he "managed a $28 million operation." It took a great deal of work to persuade him that making pegboards for the Occupational Therapy department of his local hospital was an invaluable service.

Widowhood and Widowerhood

One stark truth about a lasting marriage is that it usually means widowhood. Women still outlive men by about two to one. To outline a plan or suggest guidelines for the role change necessitated by the death of a spouse is impossible. The transition is painful and slow and sometimes incomplete. Psychologically, some women are never widowed. For example, a widow may continue to do things around the house the way her husband liked them done, talk about him as if he were still there, and remain in the same dwelling because she and her husband were very happy there. Being widowed changes other roles and precipitates crises as the widow struggles to adjust. A woman may lose not only a husband and lover but her closest companion and best friend. Even in the stormiest of unions, one grows accustomed to a spouse "for better or for worse." The loss of that spouse is devastating.

When someone is the first person in a peer group to lose a mate, he or she is somewhat socially isolated for a while. The group as a whole needs time to recover from the loss. The strength of relationships within that group determines the new role of the surviving spouse. Even in the most loyal circle of married friends, the widow or widower at times is bound to feel like the "fifth wheel on the wagon."

Widowhood is more difficult to adjust to when a woman has made a husband and his needs the focal point of her life. The reverse is also true. Loss of a spouse may mean more dependence on grown children or grandchildren to help with those things the marriage partner usually did. For example, a son may assume responsibility for house repairs for his widowed mother.

With time, the widow finds she has a social support system of other widows and even though she does not find another spouse, she is able to build a fulfilling life. The widower, if he does not remarry, is less likely to find a support group. In any case, the transition to widowhood or widowerhood is highly individualized since the most intimate of one-to-one relationships has ended.

Marriage

Remarrying or marrying for the first time in later life takes tremendous courage and readjustment. The habits and patterns of a lifetime need review and, perhaps, drastic overhauling. For two older persons to be successful in the role of newlyweds, it is helpful if they know each other quite well, are well adjusted to other roles of aging, have the approval of people they care about, and have the means to live comfortably.

Grandparenting

No matter what one says about the prospect of becoming a grandparent, or how much one may not want to be that "old," grandparenting seems to be the job nearly everyone enjoys (Fig. 5 – 5). Grandparent types are as diverse as older people are different from one another. In the first place, a vast number of them are in early middle age and are still employed. Older grandparents or great-grandparents may live in the same town they always did, or move around with the changing climate, or just travel. The character changes; the role remains the same. A grandparent is usually someone who gives unconditional love and is able to build a unique relationship with each grandchild. In this role, one discovers he is able to be the trusting, patient, playful person he wanted to be as a parent but did not have the time or energy to be.

Two factors complicate the grandparent's role in today's society. One

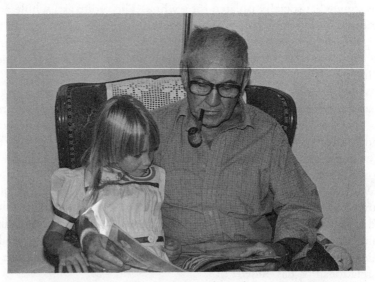

Figure 5 – 5. Grandparenting is a role nearly everyone enjoys.

is divorce. Grandparents may be called upon to give extra emotional support to the child who is torn by feelings resulting from divorce of his or her parents, while being in need of support themselves. Distance is another factor. In this mobile society, grandparents may not see their grandchildren as often as they would like because they live in different towns. Being a grandparent may be an ongoing exercise in communication, in order to relate to little people one only sees a couple of times each year. The availability of classes and workshops in grandparenting, as well as at least one regular publication, acknowledge the importance of the role.

Support Roles

Any older person can find an opportunity to play the role of support person, if not to a spouse, grandchild, or other family member, then to someone in the neighborhood or apartment building. Allowing oneself to be the "granny" or "gramps" of the neighborhood is accepting old age gracefully and having the satisfaction of being able to dole out advice, cookies, or tomatoes from the garden and to receive love and friendship in return.

Being Good at Being Old

A very old physician told a nurse who asked him why he was selling his splendid colonial style home, "I've had a long and good life. Now I will be content with enough to eat, a warm body next to mine at night, and my grandchildren to play with." People who adjust to old age know what is right for *them*.

In their book, *Enjoy Old Age*, B.F. Skinner, a behavioral psychologist, and M. Vaughan, an expert on aging, offer some common-sense advice on problem solving and tips on self-development for a happy old age. They stress the importance of keeping in touch with the past and the present and with one another. A whole chapter is devoted to the interesting idea of improving one's ability to *think* in old age.

Implications for Nursing

General Nursing Approach

The average old person whom the nurse encounters has already coped with a significant amount of stress just getting to old age. In a hospital setting, that older patient is in a situation that will generate more stress and may require some major adjustments. Given the knowledge of treatment and care the nurse has, it is tempting to approach older patients as if they should consider themselves fortunate that health care is at such a high level. The intent is to foster a positive attitude. However, failure to recognize the individual's viewpoint may foster resentment instead.

For example, today's open heart operation may indeed make it possible for a 69-year-old man to be "up and around in no time." But if that man has just learned that his 40-year-old daughter has breast cancer and if his 72-year-old brother depends on him for transportation, this fact will not matter. He may not be consoled by instruction on the technological advances in medicine, regardless of what they mean to his prognosis. Right now he is depressed about his daughter and worried about how his brother will get where he needs to go while he is recuperating. Perhaps this patient will need to talk or ask questions about cancer treatment. Perhaps someone will need to be in contact with his brother.

Careful attention to the collection of psychosocial history on admission will help the nurse identify some of the fears, sorrows, and anxieties due to the adjustments and struggles that have occurred in an older patient's life. The stress created by hospitalization is reduced by sensitivity on the part of the nurse. A patient's needs for instruction and information are also identified, and meeting these needs further reduces stress.

Signs of Psychosocial Problems

A number of complaints may be signs of psychosocial distress:

- Sleep disturbances, including difficulty in falling asleep and waking up frequently during the night
- Boredom
- Memory impairment — "Don't remember," could mean "Don't want to remember"
- Difficulty smiling, laughing, or having fun
- Regression — an older person may cope with illness and dependency by a reluctance to do simple activities of daily living without help or advice; for example, "Should I get dressed now?" or "I can't feed myself." This behavior should not be mistaken for refusal to cooperate or for senility.
- Changes in bodily functions are often normal signs of aging and *can* be symptoms of disease. It is important to recognize that such changes can also be signs of psychosocial problems. Examples of these are nausea and vomiting, diarrhea, constipation, shortness of breath, palpitations, headaches, or fatigue.

Promoting Self-Esteem

A nurse promotes self-esteem by interacting with a total personality. Who was this old woman when she was young? Did she teach school for years and take care of her father and mother? Does her ethnic background provide clues to her behavior? What were the joys of her life? The sorrows? Where was she last week at this time? What could she do?

Every day is valuable, especially when one is old. The nurse should communicate to the older person that she understands this fact. In a nursing home, for example, an aged person should be encouraged to dress every day. In the hospital, the nurse must set realistic goals for one step at a time. Respect for the older patient's input and opinions will indicate to them that the nurse is really interested in exactly *who* is in that aging body.

Summary

Old age should bring a sense of fulfillment or completion. How one arrives at old age is affected by prior personality development. Psychosocial adjustment involves learning to deal with loss. Loss of health, home, job, finances, self-esteem, and loved ones can all be part of growing old. Roles change and the transition can be traumatic, for instance, in becoming a retiree when one has maintained an identity only through a job.

Preretirement planning, returning to some kind of work, volunteering, good use of leisure time, and taking advantage of available learning opportunities are ways to ensure happy adjustment to old age. Being a grandparent or a support person for other people can be rewarding. Older people who are alone — that is, widowed, divorced, or single — often face difficult times. The nurse should be familiar with the physical and mental signs of psychosocial distress. She should be aware that older persons need to make every day count, and that treating each one as an individual will promote self-esteem.

Activities

1. Choose a family member who is over 65 "to accompany you to another planet to help with a new colony." List the reasons for your choice.
2. Ask an older person to describe the following:
   a. what good health means to them
   b. what causes stress in their life

3. Think about your older relatives and list the losses in their lives.
4. Describe what you plan to do when you retire.
5. Ask a grandparent to describe for you three joys of grand-parenting.
6. Identify an old man and an old woman with whom you are well acquainted. Make a list of specific ways in which you can help them further to develop or to maintain a positive self-image.

Bibliography

Burnside I: Psychosocial Nursing Care of the Aged, 2nd ed. New York, McGraw-Hill, 1980

Carnevali D, Patrick M (eds): Nursing Management for the Elderly, 2nd ed. Philadelphia, JB Lippincott, 1986

Dychtwald K: Wellness and Health Promotion for the Elderly. Rockville, MD, Aspen, 1986

Ebersole P, Hess P: Toward Health Aging. Human Needs and Nursing Response, 2nd ed. St. Louis, CV Mosby, 1985

Fromer M: Community Health Care and the Nursing Process, 2nd ed. St. Louis, CV Mosby, 1983

Gioiella E, Bevil C: Nursing Care of the Aging Client. Promoting Healthy Adaptation. Norwalk, CT, Appleton Century Crofts, 1985

Gress L, Bahr R Sr: The Aging Person. A Holistic Perspective. St. Louis, CV Mosby, 1984

Griffiths E: No sex please, we're over 60 . . . sexual behavior in elderly. Nurs Times 84:34–35, 1988

Hogstel M: Older widowers: a small group with special needs. Geriatr Nurs 6:24–26, 1985

National Assoc. for Home Care: Caring. Vol. 6, No. 9, Washington, DC, 1987

Schaughnessy J: Preretirement planning and the role of the occupational health nurse. AAOHN J 36:70–75, 1988

Sigman J: 50 Reasons to Get Out of Bed in the Morning. Manitowoc, WI, RP Publishers, 1987

Skinner B, Vaughan M: Enjoy Old Age: Living Fully in Your Later Years. New York, Warner Books, 1983

Steinberg F (ed): Care of the Geriatric Patient in the Tradition of E. V. Cowdry, 6th ed. St. Louis, CV Mosby, 1983

Yurick A, Spier B, Robb S, et al: The Aged Person and the Nursing Process, 2nd ed. Norwalk, CT, Appleton Century Crofts, 1984

6

Common Problems Related to Aging: Nursing Implications

Learning Objectives

When you complete this chapter, you should be able to:

1. *Identify possible problems related to aging in any completed admission interview from an older patient.*
2. *Give examples of six nursing actions and two common problems of aging that each action could help prevent or alleviate.*
3. *List six tips that will help family members prevent an older relative from falling.*

Although many problems related to aging can be identified, most of them can be managed or prevented. Disability and discomfort can often be avoided. Illness and immobility can aggravate these problems, and the opposite is true. For example, constipation is common in aging and tends to be more severe when an older person is sick and immobile. On the other hand, constipation can make an immobile person even more immobile.

Some problems are the same as symptoms of disease or are contributing factors to a nursing diagnosis. For instance, the problem of back pain can be a symptom of the disease, multiple myeloma. In a nursing diagnosis of "Altered respiratory function: ineffective airway clearance," the problem of the aged person's ineffective cough can be a contributing factor.

Because these problems are common to normal aging, they are often part of the total picture of a *well* older person. For this reason, the nurse must be familiar with them and know how to prevent injury or disease that could occur because of them. In health care settings, this knowledge must be applied in direct patient care and in teaching those who will care for the older person at home. Wellness promotion in older persons includes instruction in self-care and safe living that incorporates this knowledge (see Chap. 8).

A problem may result from more than one aging change. For example, fatigue may be caused by reduced efficiency in the respiratory system and decreased cardiac output. Therefore, the information presented in the following pages will be limited to the nursing approach to specific problems.

Just as the rate of normal aging varies from person to person, the number and types of problems that develop in each aging person also vary. All age-related problems provide a challenge for the older person who must cope with them and for those who are responsible for that person's well-being.

In some instances, there is a fine line between an actual problem and a physical finding with potential for causing trouble. One example of this is a "pot belly." Another example is the presence of certain skin lesions, like "tags" on the face and neck (see Chap. 7).

The problems selected for the Nursing Guidelines that follow are most likely to cause discomfort or dysfunction in older adults, especially when they become ill or immobile. These problems can also increase the patient's susceptibility to complications that affect recovery or rehabilitation. For example, a patient who has a cholecystectomy is reluctant to cough postoperatively for fear of precipitating pain. When that patient is elderly and has an ineffective cough, pneumonia is a serious threat. The nurse must take the common problems of aging into account when making assessments, planning, and developing care plans and teaching strategies.

Nursing Guidelines: Management of Common Problems Related to Normal Aging

1. Problem: Gradual confusion and short-term memory loss

Nursing Approach	*Family Teaching*
A. Introduce yourself each time you interact with the patient.	Make certain the older person always knows who is caring for or talking to him.
B. Keep all instructions simple and allow time for repetition.	Keep all instructions simple and repeat often.
C. Do one thing at a time. For example, the lab should not draw blood while a bath is in progress. Bathing or combing the hair should not be done while the patient is on the bedpan, commode, or toilet.	Do one thing at a time when caring for the older person, and explain everything that is happening.
D. Tell the patient everything that is happening, even if he does not seem alert enough to understand.	
E. *Sudden* confusion is not normal. When it occurs, do appropriate assessment for infection, dehydration, drug toxicity, cerebrovascular accident, and transient ischemic attack, and notify physician.	Report any sign of *sudden* confusion to the nurse.

2. Problem: Decreased sensations of pain, pressure, heat or cold

A. Regularly observe any traumatized area, such as a bruised leg, bony prominences, and other pressure points. Common sites for problems include elbows, iliac crests, coccyx, heels, and buttocks.	Routinely check any "sore" spots on the person's body, and look for redness of skin over the bony parts and pressure spots. This can be done when moving or turning. Check the areas that were resting against the mattress, cushion, or pillows. For example, when moving the person from chair to bed, observe for redness on the buttocks.

Nursing Approach

B. Frequently change patient's position.

C. A special mattress ("egg crate" foam rubber, alternating pressure, etc.) is helpful in preventing skin breakdown.

D. When giving the patient something to hold, be sure the patient has a firm grasp on the object before you release yours.

E. Be certain the patient can feel feet touching the floor before initiating any movement from bed or chair.

F. Use hot and cold applications with great care. Cover icebags and heating pads securely and with towel-thickness coverings. Check skin every three hours.

Family Teaching

Because a bedridden person cannot always feel the pain caused by pressure, he or she needs to have frequent position changes.

A foam rubber mattress is helpful in protecting skin.

Be sure the older person has a firm grip on an object (cup handle, glass, etc.) before you let go.

Be sure when you help the aged person up and down or in or out of bed to ask if he can *feel* feet touch the floor.

Cover icebags and heating pads with extra-thick pads. Check the skin every three hours. Older persons are easily burned, and their skin is easily damaged from cold.

3. Problem: Insomnia

A. Establish H.S. routine based on "what works" for the patient, such as warm milk, music, prayers, meditation, favorite pillows, or blankets from home.

B. Avoid stimulation in the evening (*i.e.*, caffeine, exercise). Coffee, tea, or hot chocolate may be part of an established routine; otherwise do not suggest these drinks. Gentle movement of joints may be helpful if the patient complains of stiffness.

C. Avoid using drugs to induce

Plan bedtime routines with older person according to what he (you) know has worked.

Avoid caffeine in the evening unless the person is accustomed to having it. Help him gently move hands, arms, feet, and legs in all directions if he feels stiff. This can be relaxing. A quiet hour before bedtime is a good idea.

Avoid sleeping pills or other drugs

Nursing Approach

sleep. When PRN sedatives have been ordered, try suggested nursing measures first.

D. Promote general comfort.

E. If naps are needed, schedule them to establish a sleep–awake pattern.

F. If treatments are necessary at night, schedule them together to reduce number of times patient needs to be awakened.

Family Teaching

for sleep. They often cause confusion and restlessness or depress the respiratory system.

Comfortable people fall asleep more easily.

If naps are needed, they should be at the same time every day.

Try not to interrupt the person's sleep.

Older persons may wake up frequently during the night. This is normal, but it also means that when they *are* sleeping it is best not to disturb them.

4. Problem: Tremors or repetitive movements

A. Assess patient's ability to do self-care and to eat independently. Provide assistance and get special equipment PRN.

May need help with self-care and eating. Get eating utensils and other things, like combs, that are easy to hold (Fig. 6–1). Check with suppliers of home health items. Put things in easy reach.

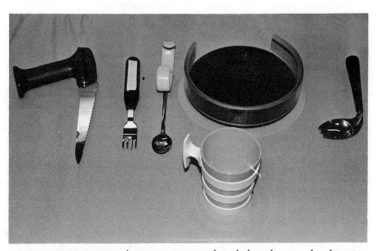

Figure 6–1. Common, adaptive eating utensils include a plate guard and suction pad to keep plate from slipping, and easy-to-grab utensils and cup.

Nursing Approach	*Family Teaching*
B. Adapt routines or environment whenever possible (*e.g.*, fill drinking glass only half full; put things within easy reach).	Try various drinking glasses to find one that the person can hold securely. Only fill the glass half full of any liquids.
C. Prevent fatigue by allowing enough time for procedures.	Take enough time to do activities and routines so older person does not get fatigued.

5. Problem: Decreased reaction time and reflexes.

A. Allow ample time for all activities and routines in which patient participation is necessary.	An older person cannot do things as fast or answer as quickly as he would like to. Take time and patience.

6. Problem: Orthostatic or postural hypotension

A. Allow patient to move slowly when getting up to avoid dizziness. Offer assistance.	Stay near the older person when he is getting up.
B. Check B.P. if dizziness occurs.	Allow him to get up slowly to avoid dizziness due to a drop in blood pressure. The person should sit on the edge of the bed for a few minutes before standing up. This is a good time to suggest that he take a few deep breaths.
	Always offer to help.

7. Problem: Delayed wound healing

A. Vigilantly observe and care for any wound.	Check any healing wound regularly, and if redness or drainage is present, notify nurse.
B. Promote good nutrition.	Proper nutrition will aid healing.

8. Problem: Increased risk of pressure sores

A. Perform routine skin care and observation of all points.	Rub powder into back, buttocks, heels, and all bony areas; if person is bedridden, do this several times a day, and more often if skin becomes reddened.
B. See 2B and 2C.	See 2B and 2C.

Nursing Approach	*Family Teaching*

9. *Problem:* Dry skin

A. Rule out malnutrition and dehydration. See 21E and 24A.

Offer liquids that the aging person *likes* to drink 5–6 times a day.

B. Encourage adequate fluid intake, *patient's choice*, when possible.

C. Use soap on skin sparingly and no alcohol. Evaluate necessity for daily bath. A complete bath may be required once a week with a partial bath daily.

Bathe only when necessary — use little soap, no alcohol. Special cleansing bars for dry skin are available at the drugstore.

D. Use humidifier PRN.

Run a cold humidifier periodically in the room where the person spends most time.

10. *Problem:* Intolerance to cold

A. Keep the patient's room at 70°F or above if indicated by his response.

Keep temperature of the older person's room at 70°F.

B. Offer extra blankets at bedtime.

"Bundle" him up at his request with extra blankets or clothing. Lightweight flannel blankets are often more comfortable than sheets next to the skin.

C. When the patient goes to other departments, take or send an extra blanket along.

11. *Problem:* Decreased ability to see

A. Be sure the patient has eyeglasses when and where needed.

Be sure the person has proper glasses.

B. Evaluate vision with eyeglasses.

Provide clear pathways in the home. Have night-lights in hallways and bathroom. Rooms should be well lit, that is, have ceiling lights and table or floor lamps.

C. Check the patient's ability to read and to distinguish be-

All pastel colors are hard to tell apart. Reds, oranges, and yel-

Nursing Approach	**Family Teaching**
tween colors, and use this information in preparing teaching sheets for taking medication at home.	lows are usually easier to see than greens, blues, and violets. This must be considered when arranging any pills for the person to take independently. Marking pill cups by "time to take" is better than referring to colors at all.
D. Keep items the patient needs to see in field of vision.	Aging persons often need things "right in front of them" to see them.
E. Provide adequate light when needed, but remember: the patient may be very sensitive to glare or too much brightness.	Reduce glare as much as possible. Chief causes of glare are shiny surfaces, such as glossy floors, bright lights, and direct sunlight.
F. Use night light and leave bathroom light on at night if the patient gets up independently.	

12. Problem: Dry eyes

A. Use artificial tear eyedrops PRN.	There are many brands of nonprescription eyedrops for "tears." Ask the pharmacist for any suggestions. Instilled several times a day or as needed, they provide much relief.

13. Problem: Impaired hearing, especially of high-frequency sounds and distinguishing between consonants

A. Speak distinctly in normal tone of voice and allow time for response.	Loss of hearing makes one feel isolated from people. Speak clearly in normal tones and give the older person enough time to answer.
B. Face patient when speaking, eye level when possible.	Face the person when speaking, eye level when possible.
C. Check ear canals for presence of impacted cerumen.	

Nursing Approach

D. Keep background noises to a minimum.

E. If the patient has a hearing aid, be sure it is working properly.

F. Report any sudden loss of hearing to the physician.

14. Problem: Vertigo

A. Evaluate the patient's ability to get up or down and ambulate independently.

B. Ask the patient about frequency and severity of this problem and provide assistance with movements PRN

C. Consider necessity for a cane.

15. Problem: Decreased sense of smell

A. Keep the patient and bed linen odor-free. The perineal area must be kept clean and dry. Change disposable pads and drawsheets PRN.

B. Assess appetite, and assist the patient with filling out menus; confer with a dietitian PRN.

16. Problem: Decreased taste

A. See 15B.

B. Accommodate patient's likes and dislikes PRN.

17. Problem: Dry mouth and/or halitosis

A. Promote good oral hygiene. Brush teeth and use mouth-

Family Teaching

Loud noises make it hard for the older person to hear what is being said.

If the person has a hearing aid, know how to keep it in working order.

Any sudden loss of hearing should be reported to the nurse.

Some dizziness with loss of balance is normal with increasing age and may come and go.

Watch and decide exactly when and how much help the older person needs to keep his/her balance when moving around.

Encourage use of cane if the person has one.

Be sensitive to odors from or around the older person, and eliminate them as soon as possible.

Make food as appealing as you can.

See 15B.

Whenever possible, the older person should have choices in food selection.

The white coating that forms on the tongue can cause an odor.

Nursing Approach	Family Teaching
wash. The tongue, palate, and insides of cheeks must be cleaned daily with a soft brush.	The whole mouth must be cleaned with a soft brush. Regular brushing of teeth and dentures and use of mouthwash is essential.
B. Offer ice chips, mints, or hard candy, if appropriate.	Allow the older person to have ice chips, mints, or hard candy if diet and condition permit.
C. Give medications with adequate fluid to ease swallowing. Offer sips of water before and after.	Give sips of water *before* giving pills, with pills, and a few seconds after pills are swallowed. Older people need extra water or other liquid to swallow medications and food.
D. Help patients avoid "dry" food when making menu selections and encourage extra fluid choices.	Moist foods are easier to chew and swallow.

18. Problem: Poor dentition/gingivitis

A. See 17A.	See 17A.
B. Adjust diet accordingly.	Make dietary changes so chewing is easier. Tooth and gum problems can be treated and prevented. Older persons should see the dentist regularly.

19. Problem: Difficulty chewing and swallowing

A. See 17D.	See 17C.
B. Diet should consist of soft foods.	Serve mostly soft foods. Help the person eat when it seems necessary.

20. Problem: Gastric upsets (nausea, vomiting, heartburn, indigestion)

A. Normally these upsets are mild and occasional. Diet alterations and antacids are sufficient for management.	Mild stomach upsets, once in a while, are normal and can be avoided by the right diet and some antacids.

Nursing Approach

B. Complaints of stomach pain or increase in gastric upsets should be evaluated and reported to the physician.

Family Teaching

Stomach *pain* and chronic upsets are not normal, and the nurse should be notified of such.

Keep a list of foods that the older person should not or cannot eat and post on refrigerator as reminder.

21. Problem: Loose stools

A. Question the patient about his elimination pattern.
B. Check for fecal impaction.
C. Monitor intake and output.
D. Consult with a dietitian on changes in diet.

Encourage the aging person to eat foods with low residue such as cheese, hard-boiled eggs, and bananas.

E. Observe for dehydration: drowsiness, dryness of mucous membranes, elevated temperature, diminished urinary output.

If loose stools increase or persist, older person may lose too much fluid, so consult with a dietitian, if possible, or check with the nurse.

Diarrhea can cause dehydration or abnormal loss of body fluids. Note signs: "laziness," fever, dry mouth and tongue, and reduced output of urine. Call the nurse if these things are present:

If a person who has not had loose stools begins to have them, first check the rectum for hard-packed stool. Such a fecal impaction will block normal passage of stool. Use a medical rubber glove, lubricate forefinger with Vaseline, ask person to take a deep breath through mouth, and then insert finger into rectum to feel for stool. Suppository or enema may be needed.

Nursing Approach

Family Teaching

22. Problem: Constipation

A. Learn about the patient's elimination patterns, and when constipation occurs do as follows:
1. Use workable suggestions by patient in relief and prevention (*e.g.*, prune juice every morning).
2. Encourage high-fiber foods.
3. Encourage fluids, patient's choice if possible.
4. Decrease any narcotics and sedatives as these drugs slow down peristalsis.
5. Act to ensure privacy for patient on bedpan or commode, or in bathroom.

Add fiber — fresh fruit, raw vegetables, and bran — to diet daily.
1. Encourage the older person to drink more water and fruit juices.
2. Avoid laxatives or stool softeners if at all possible. Long-established habits of taking such aids are hard to break. Preparations of vegetable powder that increase bulk are preferable.
3. Sometimes constipation results when the older person does not have privacy, feels rushed, or cannot get to the toilet when the urge is present.

23. Problem: Potential for drug toxicity

A. Be familiar with signs of toxicity and interactions of drugs being given.

Have a list of "what to look for" that could mean the older person is having drug reactions, and know what and when to report to the nurse.

B. Use PRN sedatives, tranquilizers, and narcotics judiciously.

24. Problem: Malnutrition

A. Evaluate history of eating habits with present appearance and condition:
1. Check for red, beefy, swollen, shiny tongue.
2. Does the patient seem to be too thin or too pale?
3. Is there iron in the diet?

Listlessness can be a sign of malnutrition. A common and easy-to-spot sign is a swollen, shiny, beefy, red tongue.

B. Evaluate appetite daily and encourage proper eating (see Chap. 7).

Be watchful of eating habits while providing a well-balanced diet. Older people need fewer calo-

Nursing Approach

Family Teaching

ries, but the daily diet should consist of these foods: 2 servings of meat, poultry, or fish; 4 servings of bread or cereal; 2 to 4 servings of dairy products; and 4 servings of fruit or vegetables. A multivitamin tablet daily is suggested.

C. Adjust diet PRN.

25. Problem: Fatigue

A. Schedule therapies far enough apart to assure best results.

Plan activities and routines with the aging person according to what that person can tolerate. Start slowly.

B. Allow enough time to do nursing routines.

Allow plenty of time for each thing that must be done.

C. Set realistic goals for activity, based on the patient's ability.

D. Promote rest periods and a good night's sleep.

Make certain the person gets enough rest and sleep.

26. Problem: Dyspnea

A. See above.

See above.

B. Schedule deep-breathing exercises. Work at getting the patient to use his diaphragm.

Help with deep-breathing exercises — have person inhale *deeply*, hold to a count of 5, exhale. Count 5. Repeat as tolerated.

27. Problem: Ineffective cough

A. See 26B.

An older person collects phlegm in the chest because he cannot cough it up, especially when he is fairly immobile. This makes him susceptible to respiratory infections.

B. Along with deep breathing, do coughing exercise. Instruct pa-

When the person is doing deep breathing, instruct him to take a

Nursing Approach

tient to take a deep breath and then cough twice. Coughing with the tongue out makes it easier to expel air.

C. Evaluate need for respiratory support measures.

D. Auscultate lungs at least once a day.

E. Be aware that even slight elevations in temperature can signal respiratory infection.

Family Teaching

deep breath, push out his tongue, and cough twice.

When one can lie with the hips elevated on pillows so head and chest are tipped back, gravity will help drain secretions out of the chest. This is called postural drainage. It can be done for 15 minutes at a time if the person can tolerate it.

28. Problem: Hypertension

A. Monitor B.P. at regular intervals.

B. If the patient is taking medication to lower B.P. or on a special diet, assess knowledge and do appropriate teaching.

C. Identify potential stressors in the present environment and modify their effect when possible. This is done through planning, instruction, and support. For example, if the patient is frightened at the prospect of an upcoming test, make sure the instructions are adequate and the patient is not feeling "rushed."

Arrange to have the older person's blood pressure checked regularly. Know what is "normal" for him.

Be sure medications are taken as ordered. Follow any diet restrictions.

Be aware of, and prevent if possible, those things that cause stress.

Nursing Approach	**Family Teaching**

29. Problem: Susceptibility to infection

A. See 27D and 27E.	Older persons often have infections without much of a fever. Be suspicious of any rise in temperature.
B. Assist the patient with good perineal care to decrease chance of urinary infection. Use urinary catheters only if absolutely necessary.	Cleanliness of the perineal area is important to reduce chance of urinary infection.
C. Adhere strictly to wound care techniques. Routinely observe any open areas on skin.	Check any open areas on skin or healing wounds for signs of redness.
D. Practice good handwashing at all times.	Protect the older person from people with obvious infections such as colds and flu. Check into flu shots.
	Foot care beyond *simple* cutting of toenails should be done by a podiatrist.

30. Problem: Peripheral edema

A. Check lower extremities and elevate if edematous.	Elevate legs if feet or legs become swollen.
B. Teach patient to limit sodium intake with help from dietitian.	Reduce salt in diet.

31. Problem: Varicosities

A. Use elastic hose PRN.	Support hose are helpful when the older person is up. Be sure they do not roll (like garters) because they cut off circulation.
B. Observe leg position frequently. Teach the patient not to keep knees flexed for long periods of time. Keep knee gatch down.	Watch that the older person does not lie with knee bent for long periods of time.

Nursing Approach	*Family Teaching*
C. Do not put pillows under knees.	Pillows should not be "bunched" under knees.
D. Evaluate all complaints of leg pain. Consider the patient at risk for thrombophlebitis.	Report any redness in calf or leg pain to nurse.
E. Avoid massaging area of pain.	Do not massage legs when painful. Pain may indicate the presence of blood clots, and massaging may cause those clots to move into the bloodstream.

32. Problem: Urinary frequency, urgency, nocturia

A. Offer bedpan or take the patient to bathroom every 2–3 hours during day and as tolerated to try to establish a pattern.	Consider use of commode that can be kept close to the person at all times to avoid fatigue from trips to bathroom.
B. Check abdomen regularly for bladder distension, indicating retention with overflow.	Feel abdomen about once a day and question older person about feeling of fullness or pressure. Report to nurse.
C. If the patient gets up independently at night, leave bathroom light on and instruct the patient to use call light, so output and habits can be monitored.	Leave night lights where necessary so the person can make safe trips to bathroom or commode.
D. For a bedridden patient, check every three hours. If awake, offer bedpan.	If using a bedpan, check every three hours. You may be able to establish some kind of routine by writing down what and when the person drinks and when he urinates. This may help you know when to offer pan.
E. Offer fluids as desired, with the exception of caffeine drinks.	Limit caffeine drinks in the evening, but encourage other fluids.

Nursing Approach	*Family Teaching*

33. Problem: Stress incontinence or dribbling of urine

A. Pad PRN. Check pads every 3 hours and change if wet. Clean and dry perineal area thoroughly. This routine must be done every 2 hours if odor or irritation is present.

Provide the older person with disposable pant liners. If this person is bedridden, change liners often, and keep padded area clean and dry.

B. Offer bedpan on a 3-hour schedule for the patient on bed rest.

C. Observe for signs of urinary infection, cloudy, foul-smelling urine, pain, burning, bleeding, and elevated temperature.

Report a fever, even a slight one, pain, bleeding, or burning on urination, and foul-smelling urine to nurse.

34. Problem: Difficulty starting urinary stream, or retention

A. See 33C.

See 33C.

35. Problem: Sexuality or self-image concerns

A. Attention-getting behavior such as expressed feelings of worthlessness and increased dependency may be clues that the older patient needs reassurance that he is not undesirable company.

An older person who suddenly seems to want more attention, or acts helpless, may be looking for reassurance that he or she is still viewed by others as an important man or woman.

B. Promote positive self-image. For example, compliment the patient on appearance, help the patient to look his or her best, hold hands, hug, or touch arm or shoulder when interacting—whatever seems appropriate. Approach the patient in a caring manner, as you would a friend.

Whatever your relationship to this older person, it is important for you to demonstrate by words and actions that you consider that person a worthwhile being, and a "fine-looking" man or woman. Helping the older person to be independent when possible will increase his or her self-esteem.

Nursing Approach	**Family Teaching**
C. Promote self-care and independence.	
D. Address the patient as he or she wishes to be addressed.	

36. Problem: Back pain.

A. Evaluate any complaints of back pain. Consider frequent back rubs, firmer mattress, physical therapy.	Provide frequent back rubs and firm mattress.
B. Report to physician PRN.	Report persistent pain to nurse.

37. Problem: Decreased range of motion, stiffness, crepitus in joints

A. Allow adequate time for the patient to do things.	Allow the older person plenty of time to do things.
B. Reposition PRN.	Help person to change position when joints feel stiff.
C. Promote range-of-motion exercises BID. Assist the patient as necessary.	Encourage movement of arms and legs regularly, in all directions.
D. Promote adequate rest.	Encourage adequate rest.
E. Evaluate need for assistive device.	

38. Problem: Weakness

A. See 37A and 37E.	See 37A.
B. Evaluate need for and give assistance PRN.	Be sure the older person has assistance as needed to do any moving around.

39. Problem: Gait problems

A. See 37E.	An aging person who has any problems with walking may need a cane or walker. Shoes or slippers should have nonskid soles and low heels. See 38B.
B. See 38B.	Remove any scatter rugs in places where the older person has to walk.

Nursing Approach	**Family Teaching**
C. Apply a safety (or gait) belt when ambulating.	A belt around the waist of the older person is essential when you walk together. You can hold on to it lightly, and it is a safety measure if he starts to fall.

40. Problem: Risk of fracture

A. See 38B and 39C.	An older person is likely to break a bone, even in a "gentle" fall. See 38B and 39A–E.
B. Leave bedrails up at all times when this patient is in bed.	
C. Keep bed in low position except when care is being given.	The bed should be low. Chairs placed against the side(s) of it at night will help prevent the person from falling out while asleep.
D. Call light should be within the patient's reach.	

Psychological Considerations

Negative feelings, such as depression and paranoia, can be symptoms of an inability to cope with normal aging. They can also be a response to declining health, to loss, or to a change in life-style. When these feelings are transient, they are as normal in an older person as they are in anyone else. A caring and empathetic attitude is the best nursing approach. The nurse must use communication skills to try and get to the real problem. When they appear to be chronic or disabling, negative feelings may be indicative of mental disorders.

Summary

There are 40 physical problems that are common in normal aging. Many of them can also be signs and symptoms of disease, so the nurse must know what they are. Some of them can be prevented. In caring for older persons, nursing measures should be included to deal with these problems or prevent them. The patient's input is important in this process because an older person often knows "what works" for himself. Family members can be instructed in ways to cope with and to prevent problems at home. Older people can become depressed or paranoid when they are unable to cope with normal aging.

Activities

1. List the physical problems of aging that are present in one of your older relatives. How does he or she seem to cope with them?
2. Think about the place where you are living. If a 90-year-old healthy person were to occupy your bedroom, what changes would you have to make in the room and in your home in general?
3. Plan a meal for an older person with a decreased sense of taste and smell.
4. Write a week of menus for a constipated person.
5. With a fellow student as your partner, demonstrate teaching a patient how to cough and breathe deeply.
6. Write four suggestions for things to do for a patient who complains of insomnia and cannot tolerate "sleeping pills."

Bibliography

Burnside I: Nursing and the Aged. A Self-Care Approach, 3rd ed. New York, McGraw-Hill, 1988

Butler R: Care of the Elderly: Special Needs for Special People. Med Times 109:46s–54s, 1981

Ebersole P, Hess P: Toward Healthy Aging. Human Needs and Nursing Response, 2nd ed. St. Louis, CV Mosby, 1985

Henderson M: Assessing the elderly, Part 2. Altered presentations. Am J Nurs 85:1103–1106, 1985

Parsons M, Levy J: Nursing process in injury prevention. J Gerontol Nurs 13(7):36–40, 1987

Patrick M et al: Medical–Surgical Nursing, Pathophysiological Concepts. Philadelphia, JB Lippincott, 1986

Tideiksaar R: How LP/VNs can play a role in the prevention of elderly falls. J Pract Nurs 36:38–41, 1986

Yurick A, Spier B, Robb S, et al: The Aged Person and the Nursing Process, 2nd ed. Norwalk, CT, Appleton Century Crofts, 1984

7

Promoting Wellness in Aging

Learning Objectives

When you complete this chapter, you should be able to:

1. List specific ways in which regular exercise can help prevent health problems in old age.
2. Identify ways to incorporate exercise into lifestyle.
3. State three things to consider when choosing an exercise program.
4. Describe a well-balanced meal.
5. Give reasons why older people sometimes lose their appetites or have poor eating habits.
6. List the most common accidents that occur in the home.
7. Discuss the aspects of safety in the home.
8. Write six safety tips for safety outside the home.
9. Identify four common medical emergencies.
10. List signs of stress.
11. Outline a program for stress management.
12. Discuss aspects of sexuality and older adults.
13. Explain why living with chronic pain is part of wellness.

The fine art of growing old is linked to staying well. In the September, 1987, issue of the publication *Caring*, true stories about people over 100 years of age were rich with their ideas on wellness. Exercise, keeping busy, forgiving and forgetting, and staying away from doctors were some of the suggestions offered by these centenarians. Their stories imply that to stay well one must attend to the whole person: body, mind, and spirit. Definitions of wellness are personal and they change with advancing age and the onset of problems. Wellness should be the responsibility of the individual. For many older people this responsibility becomes difficult because they are either unable or reluctant to make their own decisions about what is good for them.

Self-care is one dimension of wellness, and it emphasizes fulfilling basic needs that sustain life in a safe and normal way. For an aging person the challenges are eliminating or minimizing self-care limitations and retaining control over his or her own life. The nurse helps the older person by giving the assistance or instruction that is needed.

Promoting wellness for the whole person begins with a look at what is required to keep an aging body mobile and functioning in activities of daily living. Mental health is an important component of wellness. It encompasses stress management, sexuality, usefulness, and belonging. The older person must be aware of how to create and maintain a safe environment. Being "well" is a continuous task when one has a chronic disease or pain. The spiritual aspect of wellness is highly individual. The nurse who is sensitive and open to understanding the spiritual needs of older people can learn and grow in the process. In all areas of wellness promotion, the nurse is an educator and resource person.

Wellness and Self-Care

The Meaning of Health and Wellness

Health may be defined as the absence of disease or illness or the state of having a sound mind and body. Both definitions of health imply present status only. In contrast, wellness is ongoing and is often described as a continuum. Wellness is harmony among all the components of the individual's internal and external life, including the physical body, mental processes, attitudes, emotions, and environment. The meaning of environment is broad and considers social and cultural conditions as well as where one lives. Well-being is the state of being happy, and it is part of wellness.

Regardless of where one is in the course of a lifetime, there is an optimal level of functioning. This is true for the person who must adjust to physical limitations of aging or the effects of a chronic disease. A degree of wellness is always achievable, even in the process of dying. In dying, one can attain a state of spiritual and emotional well-being.

Who is well? There is always a personal aspect in the definition of wellness. For example, let us take two 67-year-old unmarried women in totally different circumstances. One is a retired bookkeeper who has been able to invest her money well and now enjoys a fairly luxurious life-style. She owns a duplex, drives a car, and travels extensively. She has always been in excellent physical health. She has said she would be "sick" if she couldn't "come and go."

The other woman has not been employed for ten years. During some of this time, she lived with and cared for her aging mother on the money from the sale of two family farms. Now she lives in an efficiency apartment in a senior citizens apartment complex. Her only source of income is Social Security. Two years ago she was diagnosed as a diabetic and has learned to give her own insulin. Although she depends on relatives or neighbors when she needs to go out, she is a happy and contented person. She considers herself "lucky" to be as "well off" as she is.

The meaning of wellness must be modified for each individual in the presence of physical problems related to aging, psychosocial stressors such as loss or role changes, and chronic disease or discomfort.

Self-Care

Self-care means the safeguarding and sustaining of life. The ability to secure and use food, air, and water and meet the needs related to body functions, such as elimination, is essential to self-care. A balance between rest and activity that is acceptable to each person should be achieved. The older person's capacity for self-care can become limited by altered states of health, changes related to aging, socioeconomic factors, and lack of knowledge and skills. Motivation is a critical factor in self-care and may be determined by satisfaction with life, companionship, and financial status.

In promoting wellness through self-care, the nurse assesses abilities and limitations and helps the older person to adapt to the environment, to modify habits and activities, and to learn new things. Using the nursing process, the nurse identifies needs and potential problems. Nursing diagnoses are based on these data and are guidelines in teaching wellness. The following are examples of such nursing diagnoses and possible nursing actions:

DIAGNOSES	ACTIONS
1. Knowledge deficit related to exercises for older adults	Explain benefits of regular exercise. Discuss basic types of exercise and give examples or demonstrate how they can be modified or incorporated into activities of daily living (ADL).
2. Potential for altered nutrition: less than body requirements, related to decreased taste and smell	Suggest ways to make a plate of food look appetizing. Offer some simple recipes based on person's preferences in food. Suggest ways to make mealtime more enjoyable, such as having some meals in a group setting, like a senior center.
3. Activity intolerance related to discomfort from arthritis in hands	Suggest using warm cloths or soaks prior to doing tasks that are painful. Get a catalog of home health aids and point out special utensils and homemaking aids.

Wellness for an Aging Body

What Aging Does

Remember that in normal aging, the body slows down (see Chap. 3). Tissues lose elasticity and flexibility. Some function is lost because of a decrease in neurons. Walls of blood vessels thicken. In the body systems, where the work of transporting and changing fluids and other substances is carried on, the functions are less efficient. For example, a number of aging factors impair ventilation, which is the exchange of carbon dioxide for oxygen in the lungs. Reduced elasticity in the alveoli and the rigidity of intercostal muscles and cartilage are two of those factors. Since body systems are interdependent, decreased efficiency in one affects the efficiency of another. For example, arteriosclerosis, or thickening of the blood vessels, in the kidneys reduces renal blood flow and glomerular filtration. Overall, as one ages, more effort and self-discipline are necessary to maintain adequate functioning of body systems and to do those things that were once matters of routine in work or play.

An aging body may seek to "take it easy" by remaining immobile. Unfortunately, immobility is deadly. A major task in promoting wellness in older persons is to motivate them to remain active.

Becoming Sedentary

Technology has all but eliminated the everyday ways to get regular exercise in and around the home as well as the workplace. Modern appliances and riding lawnmowers have made maintenance of house and yard less strenuous. Constant improvements in machinery continue to decrease the amount of physical labor in most occupations.

The older one gets, the easier it is to become sedentary and to stay that way. Both retirement and release from the responsibility of rearing children offer persons more time for relaxation and a greater choice of activities. After years of hard work and demanding schedules, many older persons are contented with purely social activities. In fact, they may feel that they have earned the right to do so. In a sense, this is true, but it is important for them to realize that the quality of life as they grow even older is associated with maintaining health and independence. The tendency to tire easily with advancing age can become an excuse to decrease all physical activity and to resist the idea of regular exercise. Furthermore, up until now, society had never expected its older members to be physically fit.

Benefits of Regular Exercise

Remaining active in old age can be a chore. Yet exercise will help decrease and, perhaps, reverse some of the detrimental changes related to aging. Even in the presence of chronic conditions, some kind of regular exercise is recommended. There are many benefits of exercise for older people:

- Improved circulation and ventilation
- Increased muscle strength and tone
- More joint flexibility
- Thicker, stronger bones because of increased mineral content
- Decreased body fat
- Lower blood pressure
- Better glucose tolerance
- More energy
- Decreased susceptibility to depression
- Reduced tension
- Enhancement of self-image

Incorporating Exercise Into Life-style

Exercise can be successfully incorporated into an older person's life-style. This entails knowledge of what exercise is all about. Busy people often say that they do not *need* "any more exercise." Yet one can reach the point of physical exhaustion every day and maintain a desirable weight — and still develop unnecessary stiffness in joints and muscles. Healthful activity includes exercise that will help keep joints mobile, strengthen muscle groups, and improve ventilation and circulation.

Throughout activities of daily living, some simple routines can be established and habits formed that will provide beneficial exercise. Instructions for the older adult are as follows:

- When you get up in the morning, stand as tall as you can, stretch your arms straight up to the ceiling, and count to five. Then wiggle your fingers. Repeat several times.
- After stretching in the morning, take three deep breaths. Fill the chest and stomach, hold to count of three, and exhale. Push your stomach in and up toward the diaphragm as you breathe air out.
- When bathing, you can increase circulation by washing your arms from your fingertips toward your shoulders. Wash your legs from your feet up to your thighs.
- When you are doing something that does not require you to watch what you are doing, move your head from side to side, back and forth and around in a circle, stretching your neck.
- When you sit down to rest, stretch your legs and feet straight out in front of you. Then bend your feet back toward your body. Point them out once more. Feel how tight this makes your calf and thigh muscles. Repeat several times. Wiggle your toes.
- While you watch television, stretch your arms straight out to the sides and make circles with your hands, first clockwise and then counterclockwise. Then make circles with your arms, moving from the shoulders, first clockwise and then counterclockwise. Do this a couple of times. Then stretch your legs out straight and do the same thing with your feet and then your legs. Repeat a couple of times.
- While sitting, take some time to tighten your buttocks and hold to the count of five, and then tighten your abdomen and do the same.
- Every time you are going to turn a faucet on or off, stop, straighten your spine, hold your shoulders back and take a deep breath.
- Be posture-conscious — stand straight — sit straight. *Poor* posture eventually causes pain. *Good* posture helps your balance, improves muscle tone, and gives your organs room to do their work.

Older persons should be encouraged to walk. Walking strengthens muscles and bones and improves circulation. Swinging the arms and moving the fingers, and clenching and unclenching the hands, increase the benefits obtained from walking. Shopping malls are a good place to walk when weather does not permit being out of doors. In some communities, shopping malls open their main doors an hour earlier in the morning to accommodate walkers. In any community, this possibility should be investigated. Swimming, biking, or riding a stationary bicycle are good for muscle strength, and tone, and they do not stress joints.

Starting an Exercise Program

One can begin an exercise program at any age. Stories about persons who have attained physical fitness in old age appear regularly in magazines and newspapers. The nurse should be familiar with some of these accounts and use the people discussed as examples when they teach fitness. Two publications that are excellent resources for such material are *50 Plus*, published by Retirement Living Publishing Co., and *Modern Maturity*, which is published by the American Association of Retired Persons.

How does an aging person choose the right kind of exercise program? First, exercise should be enjoyable. The options are exercising alone, with a friend, or joining a group. Older people prefer groups or classes that allow for flexibility in the routines and encourage socializing. A person who chooses to exercise alone or with a friend should be encouraged to try different kinds of exercise and see how they feel. Many exercises can be modified to meet an individual's needs. For example, if lying on the floor is uncomfortable, one can sit on a chair and do many of the same movements, such as straight leg raising. Establishing fairly regular routines and times for exercise will help one stay with a program. Motivation to exercise may also be increased if the older person understands the importance of strengthening muscles to reduce strain on the joints and the back. It is important to remember that the older person who is overweight or who has been inactive for years should embark on an exercise program very slowly. A medical examination is recommended for these people and for those who have a chronic disease, disability, or are taking medication (see the display, "An Exercise Program for Older Persons").

Aerobics

An aerobic form of exercise is one that uses oxygen and is continuous. Running and walking are aerobic. The purpose of aerobic exercise is to improve the cardiovascular system. For older persons, this could mean less shortness of breath on exertion and less fatigue during physical activities. Ideally, aerobic exercise works the heart hard enough to increase its efficiency without causing undue stress. No older person should

An Exercise Program for Older Persons

Warm Up Muscles for 5 – 10 Minutes by Stretching

1. *Arms.* Stand with your feet about one foot apart. Raise your arms up as if you could touch the ceiling. Count to 10. Lower arms. Then repeat.
2. *Legs.* Stand about 2 – 3 feet behind a sturdy chair. Put your feet together and point them toward the chair. Lean your body forward as if you were doing a push-up off the back of the chair. Count to 10. Return to upright position. Then repeat.
3. *Neck.* Stand straight, arms at sides and feet about one foot apart. Tuck your chin in your chest. Slowly turn your head to the left, then roll to the back and continue to the right and circle to the front. Do this 3 times, then repeat in the opposite direction 3 times.

Exercises

1. Standing, stretch arms out in front, palms up. Bend elbows. Bring hands to touch shoulders. Make circles with the elbows by bringing them toward each other, then up, out, around, and back to the front of your body. Repeat 3 times.
2. Stretch arms out to sides, palms up. Turn palms down, then up. Repeat up, down, 5 times. Then make small circles with the hands just at the wrist. Do 10 circles forward and then 10 backward.
3. With arms still outstretched, do 10 circles using the whole arm circling forward, and then 10, circling backward.
4. With hands on the waist, bend slowly to the right and then straighten. Do this 3 times. Repeat to the left.
5. With hands on the waist, twist slowly to the right and then look as far over that shoulder as you can. Turn forward. Do this 3 times. Repeat to the left.
6. Stand straight, arms at sides, and tighten abdominal muscles. Count to 10. Repeat 3 times.
7. Sit on a chair. Raise the right leg straight out in front. Bend the foot toward your body. Count to 5. Return the foot to the floor. Repeat 3 times. Repeat with the left leg. Then do both legs together 3 times.
8. Bring the right knee up toward your chest and hug it. Count to 5. Lower the leg to the floor. Do this 3 times.

(continued)

An Exercise Program for Older Persons (*Continued*)

Exercises

      Repeat with the left leg.

9. Raise both legs, point toes straight ahead, and move the legs out to the sides. Then bring them toward each other and cross them in a scissors motion. Continue this movement to count of 10.
10. Hold the legs straight out again. Point the feet out to the sides and then turn them in. Do this 5 times.

After these exercises, walk around the room swinging your arms for 10 to 15 minutes. Cool down muscles by repeating stretching exercises.

---

do aerobic exercise without consulting a physician to learn what his individual limits are.

In a 45- to 60-minute planned "senior aerobics" session, warm-up periods with stretching and joint loosening exercises in sitting and standing positions precede the aerobic exercise. This exercise may be a brisk walk around the gymnasium while doing various arm exercises, and then doing some dancing kicks and marching steps for 15 to 20 minutes. A cool-down period similar to the warm-up follows.

Competitive Activities

Competitive events or "Senior Olympics" are becoming more popular and provide motivation for older people to achieve and maintain physical fitness. These events include a variety of activities such as shuffleboard, walking relays, golf, bean bag tosses, and volleyball. Community sponsors may be such organizations as aging agencies, the YMCA, the YWCA, bowling alleys, hospitals, and educational institutions.

Modifying Exercise

Aging persons with chronic diseases can benefit from exercising within their capabilities. Swimming and exercising in a swimming pool is excellent for the arthritic. People with chronic obstructive pulmonary disease may be advised to swim, walk, ride a bicycle, or try exercises suggested in this chapter. It cannot be emphasized too strongly that exercise programs for older persons with health problems must be tailored to individual needs and begin with medical consultation.

More Nursing Implications

Obviously, all exercise programs for older people are very similar. The nurse needs to understand the basic purposes and benefits of exercise in order to teach older people and help them make decisions about selecting the appropriate kind of group or individual activity (see the display, "Tips for Senior-Safe Exercise").

Keeping older people physically fit is a family affair. Many people are unaware of the importance of exercise in old age. Well-meaning relatives often try to make life easier for their elders instead of encouraging them to remain active. Idle hands become stiff. Simple things like allowing the older person to fasten his or her own seat belt in an automobile may be time consuming, but these activities will help the person to maintain manual dexterity. Family members should be given the same information about exercises as their older relatives so that they can be supportive while monitoring progress.

Tips for Senior-Safe Exercise

- Always start slowly and stop gradually.
- Wait at least one hour after eating before beginning any exercise.
- Balance all activity with rest.
- Exercise every other day.
- Practice normal, relaxed breathing during exercise.
- Avoid jerking, bouncing, and extreme twisting of the body.
- Listen to your body: pain means the exercise you are doing is not the right kind.
- Dizziness, shortness of breath, unusual fatigue, and excessive sweating, besides pain, are also warning signals.
- Remember that wind increases the heart's work load.
- Exercise with care in hot weather.
- Morning and evening are usually the best times for exercise.
- In cold weather, remember the "wind chill factor."
- Wear jogging shoes — they are shaped like the foot and have cushioned support.
- Remember that older bones are thinner, so falls can mean fractures.
- Exercise *does* reduce tension, but if you are extremely upset, exercise more slowly.

Special Body Care

Eyes

Cataracts and glaucoma are major eye problems in older people. A cataract is hard to ignore because the clouding of the lens impairs all vision. Glaucoma, an increase in intraocular pressure which can cause blindness, can be acute or chronic. Symptoms of acute glaucoma are severe eye pain, nausea, and vomiting. Blurred vision follows, and blindness can result within a day. The treatment is usually medication, but surgery may be performed to establish a channel to filter the aqueous fluid.

Chronic glaucoma is more common, and the symptoms develop so slowly that the affected person may not realize he is having vision problems until it is too late. Loss of peripheral vision, seeing halos around lights, and headache are the early symptoms. Impairment of central vision follows, affecting one or both eyes. The disease is incurable.

Medications that raise the blood pressure also increase intraocular pressure, so they must not be taken by or given to a person with glaucoma. Stress, tight clothing, excessive fluids, constipation, or any physical strain will increase intraocular pressure and should be avoided. Regular eye examinations are imperative to detect this disease in its early stages. Wearing a "Medic Alert" bracelet that identifies one as having glaucoma is a good idea (see Chap. 6 for more suggestions on eye care).

Ears

Periodic examination of the ears will prevent the accumulation of cerumen, or ear wax. When loss of hearing is apparent, an audiometric examination should be done before any hearing aid is purchased. This is a priority in promoting wellness. For some hearing deficits, hearing aids are useless.

Teeth and Mouth

More and more people are retaining most of their own teeth throughout life. Even for those who do not, oral health is important. The teeth and gums should be brushed thoroughly with a soft toothbrush, preferably after each meal. Flossing should be done daily. Pale gums are common in older persons because of reduced capillary blood supply. They are easily inflamed and require close and regular inspection. Dentures must be removed daily for thorough cleaning and to soak overnight.

Dentures loosen as underlying bone deteriorates, so they need periodic relining. Older persons should be encouraged to visit a dentist at least once a year (for oral hygiene suggestions, see Chap. 6).

New technology in dentistry includes the use of dental implants or replacing individual teeth. These implants are expensive, but they may be indicated for those people who have excessive problems with poorly fitting dentures or for those who can afford implants and simply want to get more enjoyment out of eating. Underbites and overbites in middle-aged persons can be corrected.

Skin

Older persons should be taught to inspect their skin when bathing. Any change in a skin lesion, such as in hardness, size, or color, must be reported to a physician. Skin lesions, such as yellowish brown warts and skin tags, are common with advancing age. They also require close observation. Skin tags can be removed if they are irritated by clothing. The tiny hemorrhagic spots known as purpura may contribute to skin breakdown in older persons who sit too long without changing position. Lanolin or a mild lotion is good on dry skin.

Breasts

Monthly breast examinations are still necessary for older women, even though they have passed menopause. Any mass or tenderness must be examined by a physician.

Varicosities

Varicose veins are common in older persons. Support hosiery may make the legs more comfortable. Walking increases circulation and reduces the "heavy feeling" in lower legs. Garters and garter belts, rolled stockings or knee-high stockings should never be worn as they may impair circulation. Tight underpants may also interfere with circulation.

Feet

Many foot problems in older persons are prevented by wearing proper fitting shoes so the toes have room to spread. Sturdy, low-heeled, rubber-soled shoes are best, and laced shoes may be safer than slip-ons. Feet should be washed and inspected daily, and it is important to dry thoroughly between the toes to prevent infection. Toenails should be trimmed straight across or filed frequently. Corns and calluses can be rubbed with a pumice stone after the feet have been soaked and softened. Aging persons must be instructed never to cut calloused skin or corns, and they should report injuries to their physician. Healing is slow in the older foot and infection is a threat.

Nutrition

Proper nutrition is essential to wellness in older persons. It helps them to stay healthy, and it contributes to the quality of life. With a few exceptions, the basic requirements for calories and nutrients do not change throughout adulthood (Fig. 7-1).

Caloric requirements are lower after age 50 and continue to decline until age 75 for two reasons. First, with aging there is a decrease in basal metabolism, or the amount of energy used by the body at rest. Second, most older persons tend to limit their physical activities. For persons aged 51 to 75, the recommended daily allowance (RDA) suggests about a 10% decrease in caloric intake; after the age of 75, the recommended decrease is 20% to 25%.

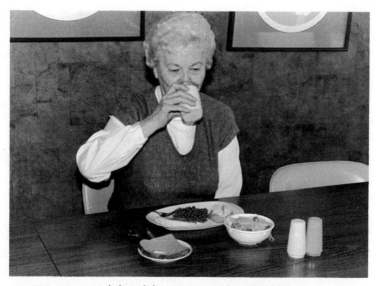

Figure 7–1. A balanced diet is necessary for good health at any age.

Protein

Proteins are the body builders, and meat, fish, poultry, eggs, and dairy products are the best sources. Although protein needs in aging have not been clearly established, one estimate for protein is 15% to 20% of total caloric intake. Chronic disease does increase the need for protein.

Carbohydrates

Heat and energy are produced by carbohydrates. About half of the daily diet should consist of this nutrient. Plant products supply the greatest amounts of carbohydrates. Fresh fruits, vegetables, and whole-grain breads and cereals are the best sources. Cellulose, or roughage, is supplied by carbohydrates and is beneficial in maintaining bowel regularity.

Fats

Fats produce twice as much heat and energy as carbohydrates, but they have more calories. Foods high in fat are butter, egg yolks, pork, and nuts. A healthful diet for an older person should be no more than about 25% fatty food.

Vitamins

Vitamins A, B-complex, C, D, E, and K have regulating functions and aid in digestion and metabolism. Vitamins also strengthen resistance to disease. They are present in sufficient quantities in a well-balanced diet.

Mineral oil is not recommended as a laxative for elderly persons. If an older adult has been taking it regularly and is reluctant to change laxatives, he or she should be instructed not to take it close to mealtime because it prevents the absorption of vitamins A, D, E, and K.

Minerals

Minerals have regulating functions and are necessary for building bones and teeth and forming red blood cells. Minerals required in the daily diet include calcium, phosphorus, iron, iodine, copper, potassium, sodium, zinc, and magnesium. Like vitamins, they are available in a wide variety of foods. Older people need additional calcium in the diet. Where 800 mg was once considered sufficient, some experts now recommend 1000 mg to 1500 mg daily for people over age 60. Calcium intake and absorption decreases with age. Osteoporosis, a metabolic bone disease which is more common in women, develops after menopause and is related to a calcium deficiency. The disease is characterized by thin, brittle bones (see the display, "Foods That Contain Calcium").

The RDA of iron decreases in old age. However, the elderly are prone to iron-deficiency anemia because of the following factors:

- Decreased meat intake due to difficulty in chewing, change in food preference, or poor economic status
- Factors that inhibit iron absorption, such as chronic use of antacids, drinking excessive amounts of tea, and reduced hydrochloric acid in gastric juice
- Chronic blood loss due to some arthritis drugs or anticoagulants

---

A List of Foods That Contain Calcium:

Major Sources—250 mg per serving	*Serving Size*
Milk (whole, 2%, 1%, skim milk)	8 ounces
Cheese (Parmesan, Swiss, ricotta)	1 ounce
Sardines (with bones)	3 ounces
High-calcium cocoa mix	1 package
Carnation Instant Breakfast drink (made with milk)	1 package

Moderate Sources—150–250 mg per serving	
Cheese (Cheddar, brick, blue, Colby, mozzarella, Limburger, American, Monterey, Edam, Muenster, provolone)	1 ounce
Cheese spread	1 tablespoon
Yogurt	½ cup
Pudding	½ cup
Custard	½ cup
Salmon (canned with bones)	3 ounces
Tofu	4 ounces
Collard greens	½ cup

(Courtesy of Bellin Hospital, Nutrition Services, Green Bay, Wisconsin)

Water

Three quarts, or 3000 ml, of water daily is required by an older person to replace fluids lost through stool, urine, perspiration, and breathing.

Causes of Nutritional Problems

Poor eating habits in an aging person may go back as far as childhood, or they may have developed for other reasons. Hurried meals and fad diets contribute to poor eating habits. Many factors influence appetite. Inadequate nutrition is possible even when an older person seems to be eating well. To promote wellness, the nurse must first understand the reasons why older people have poor eating habits and poor appetites.

Nutritional deficits and problems may be caused by aging changes, lack of exercise, drug therapy, chronic disease, or psychosocial factors.

Aging Changes

A review of the common problems related to aging will help the nurse recall changes that interfere with eating and digestion (see Chap. 6). Loss of taste and smell, dental problems and dry mouth may diminish an older person's desire to eat in the first place. When someone who always believed that meat makes the meal loses the capacity for chewing steak or roast, he may prefer not to eat meat in any form. Adjustment of the diet to compensate for this loss of protein may not occur to him. Decreased peristalsis and decreased gastric secretions may mean intolerance to longtime favorite foods. Fear of an upset stomach, diarrhea, flatulence, or constipation increases a reluctance to eat many foods that are sources of essential nutrients. People who have nocturia, dribbling, or other problems with urinary continence may be reluctant to drink water.

Lack of Exercise

An older person may consider toast and pudding a substantial meal because he "did not work hard enough to get very hungry." He may be unaware that satisfying hunger is not the same as taking adequate nourishment.

Drug Therapy

Some medications affect the appetite or cause constipation. Laxatives reduce the absorption of nutrients.

Chronic Disease

Arthritis in the upper extremities may limit the older person's ability to prepare food. People who have diabetes or hypertension or other chronic diseases often have dietary restrictions that affect the appetite.

Psychosocial Factors

The following statements highlight some of the psychosocial factors that influence the nutrition of older adults:

"It's too much trouble to cook for one person."
"It's no fun eating alone."
"I can't get to the store like I want to."
"Meat and produce are too expensive."
"It's hard to buy for one person."

Social isolation due to the death of a spouse, relatives, or close friends causes depression and may decrease the appetite and influence eating habits. Snacking on toast or crackers may replace eating meals. Older people may develop poor eating habits when they feel useless or bored.

Lack of transportation prohibits trips to the supermarket. An older person who is dependent on others to purchase his groceries, or on a store that delivers groceries, cannot take advantage of sales. This can be expensive. Retirement budgets put limits on what one can spend for food. For the older person who lives in a room without cooking facilities, eating out is a real financial strain.

Promoting Proper Nutrition

An older person may be more interested in his own nutrition when he knows what it should be. Selections from the basic four food groups are necessary every day (Fig. 7-2): meat, fish, and poultry (two servings); cereals and breads (four servings); fruits and vegetables (four servings); and dairy products (two servings). Six to eight glasses of water are essential. Food preferences are strong by the time one reaches old age. They are influenced by tradition, values, and ethnicity and may be an obstacle when they do not include adequate nutrients.

Dietary modifications can be suggested to meet special needs of this age group. For instance, as people get older they benefit from additional fiber in the diet as a means to prevent constipation. Whole grains are an excellent source of fiber. An older adult should be advised to eat whole-grain breads rather than breads made from refined flour. Many people

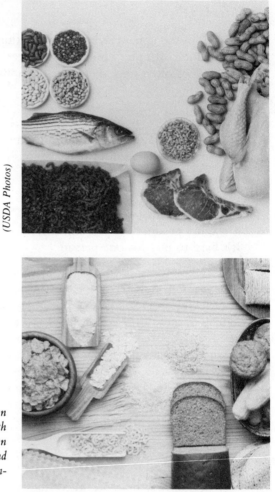

Figure 7–2. Nutrients play an important role in the normal health of an older person. (Eschleman MM: Introductory Nutrition and Diet Therapy, p. 41. JB Lippincott, Philadelphia, 1984)

rely on stewed fruit or fruit juices for bowel regularity. This is a very individualized aspect of wellness, and the nurse who is helping an aging person with menu planning must take this into consideration. When one cannot chew or digest fresh fruits and vegetables, they should be cooked or blended into drinks. Meat can be ground or chopped in a blender. Excessive salt should be avoided.

Powdered milk added to regular milk or sprinkled in scrambled eggs and casseroles will provide calcium and add protein to the diet, replacing some meat. Since many older adults do not drink enough milk, finding additional sources of calcium is a priority. Cheese is excellent, but it is high in fat and, for some people, cheese is constipating.

Lay publications give much attention to the subject of calcium supple-

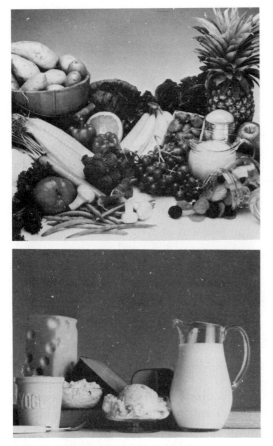

(*Fig. 7–2 continued*)

ments for aging people, especially women. To prevent osteoporosis, physicians commonly prescribe the combination of calcium carbonate, oral estrogen, and exercise for postmenopausal women. The progression of the disease can be slowed down or halted by this treatment.

Are vitamin and mineral supplements generally necessary? A well-balanced diet contains all requirements for nutrients. Vitamin quackery is practiced on the older person, particularly in the treatment of arthritis and impotence. It is not uncommon for an older person to be taking a multivitamin plus one or two other vitamin preparations because he has heard or read somewhere that they are helpful. When a person with arthritis is taking a certain vitamin and the disease happens to go into remission, probably nothing will convince him that he is not being helped by that preparation. Instruction about the purposes of vitamins and the dangers of overdose is the best course of action open to the nurse (see Table 7-1). Vitamin and mineral supplements should not and cannot take the place of food. Since their use is potentially dangerous, the older person should seek the advice of a physician before taking *any* vitamins or minerals.

Obesity

Weight control is usually harder as one grows older, yet it is a prerequisite for a long, healthy life. Women are more prone to obesity in later years than men. There is a tendency to develop a pot belly and to accumulate fat on the hips and thighs in old age. Fat around the midsection puts a considerable strain on the back muscles. A low-fat, low-sodium diet along with reduced caloric intake will be beneficial to the older person who is struggling with the problem of weight control.

Shopping Suggestions

Cost is frequently the determining factor in an older person's selection of food. A nurse can offer these suggestions to help an older person stretch food dollars:

- Buy large cans, jars, or packages if they are the best buy and split the food and the cost with a friend.
- When you do buy just for yourself, buy single-serving cans of vegetables and soups instead of leaving unused portions of bigger cans in the refrigerator to spoil.
- Check generic brands. They may be the same as name brands and cost less.
- If you have freezer space, buy large bags of frozen vegetables and fruits and cook or thaw only as much as you need.
- Freeze meat in one-serving packages. Meat, especially ground meat, should not be left in the refrigerator uncooked for more than two days.
- If you are watching your weight, remember that many "dietetic" products contain as many calories as those made from regular ingredients and are often more expensive.

Reading Labels

Older persons may not be able to read all the small print on cans and boxes. They should be taught to ask questions of clerks when they are concerned about contents, for instance, salt and sugar. Labels list ingre-

Table 7-1. For Older Adults: Simple Facts about Vitamins

Vitamins	Sources	What it Does	Harmful Effects of Overdose
Vitamin A	Dark green and yellow-orange vegetables; yellow-orange fruit (peaches); dairy products	Helps you to have healthy skin and eyes; helps resist infection	Headaches, nausea, vomiting, double vision, ringing in ears, dry skin, hair loss, pain in muscles, joints, abdomen, brittle nails, anemia, enlarged spleen
Vitamin B-1 (thiamine)	Meat, especially pork, liver; enriched or whole-grain cereal, bread; eggs; dried beans, peas, soybeans, potatoes, broccoli	Good for digestion; keeps nervous system healthy, less irritable; helps body release energy	Probably none*
Vitamin B-2 (riboflavin)	Milk, cheese, ice cream, enriched or whole-grain bread, cereal; meat (liver is best), fish, eggs, poultry	Keeps eyes, skin, mouth, healthy; helps body produce energy	Unknown
Niacin	Peanut butter, beans; lean meat, especially liver, fish, poultry; milk; enriched or whole-grain bread and cereal	Good for nervous system, digestion, skin, mouth and tongue; helps body use food	Tingling sensation; flushed skin; liver damage
Vitamin B-6 (pyridoxal)	Gland meats, (kidneys, liver); whole-grain bread and cereals	Helps body use protein	Probably none*
Folic acid	Green vegetables; whole wheat; fish, liver; dairy products; eggs	Helps body use protein; part of body tissues and red blood cells	Probably none*

(continued)

Table 7-1. (*Continued*)

Vitamins	Sources	What it Does	Harmful Effects of Overdose
Vitamin B-12	Red meat; same foods as folic acid	Helps body use protein—needed to make red blood cells	Probably none*
Vitamin C (ascorbic acid)	Citrus fruits (oranges, lemons, grapefruits, limes); strawberries, cantaloupe; white potatoes, tomatoes, green peppers, broccoli, cabbage, raw greens	Helps make connective tissue; used in healing and in fighting infection; good for bones, teeth, blood vessels; helps other body functions	Kidney stones, gout
Vitamin D	Sunshine; vitamin D milk; fish liver oils	Helps body use calcium; good for bones	Nausea, lack of appetite, weight loss, hardening of soft tissue; kidney damage
Vitamin E	Wheat germ; margarine; egg yolk; green leafy vegetables	Helps with fat digestion; keeps body cells healthy	Thins blood; may cause hemorrhage
Vitamin K	Cereal; green leafy vegetables; fruit; liver; margarine, soybean oil	Important for normal blood clotting—to stop bleeding	Anemia

*This does *not* mean one can take large amounts safely—what is not too much for one person may be too much for another.

dients contained by amounts in descending order. Labels also provide information about the nutrients in the whole container and in single servings. Dates stamped on containers and wrappings should be checked because they indicate freshness.

Preparing and Serving Food

Using fat or flour in the preparation of food adds unnecessary calories. Vegetables should not be overcooked or steamed too long because they lose vitamin and mineral content. Herbs vary the taste of food when one must limit salt and pepper.

Eating alone is something many older people are forced to do a lot of the time, and it can be lonely. These are suggestions the nurse can offer to the older person to make meals for one more enjoyable:

- Arrange to eat meals when *you* want to, and if more and smaller meals suit you better than three larger ones, that should be your habit.
- Set a pretty table with good dishes.
- If you enjoy watching television, reading, or listening to the radio while you eat, do so.

Sharing a meal with others can be much more pleasant and relaxing than eating alone. The National Program for Older Americans has established nutrition projects throughout the country to provide well-balanced, low-cost meals for people age 65 and older. Nutrition sites may be in senior centers, community centers, churches, and other locations. For example, a program may be set up to serve a hot meal every weekday at noon. Participants in the meals are asked to pay only if they can, and only what they can afford. Often, older persons will know about these meals, but they will be reluctant to go alone or accept a "handout." The opportunity for meeting friends can be as beneficial as the meal, and it is from this standpoint that the nurse can make the suggestion.

Food Stamps

A limited income may qualify an older person for food stamps. These enable the person who buys them to get more food for less money. The social stigma attached to the use of food stamps may deter someone in need from using them. Some older persons do not know they are available or how to apply for them. This can be tactfully mentioned in any general instruction on nutrition.

Safety

For an older person to experience high-level wellness, that person must feel safe. Areas to consider in discussing safety are conditions in and around the home, driving a car, taking medications, knowledge of first aid, and protection against crime.

Safety in the Home

Accidents in the home cause almost half of the injuries fatal to the elderly. Most fatal accidents happen in the bedroom, although many serious hazards can be found in the bathroom. These accidents are falls, fire, suffocation and posioning. Numerous nonfatal injuries occur in the home, mostly in the kitchen. Many of these accidents could have been prevented.

Falls by older persons are a frequent occurrence, and some of them can not be prevented. For example, getting up at night with the urgent need to void may cause an older person to hurry to the bathroom. Dizziness from postural hypotension due to an abrupt change in position may make that person fall.

Age-related changes such as irregularity in gait cause falls. Diminished color and depth perception, decrease in acuity and peripheral vision, and the ability to recover from glare are responsible for numerous falls. Chronic conditions and reactions to medications are common sources of dizziness. Fear of falling can cause one to become easily startled and then fall.

Those falls that might be prevented often result from a lack of safety features or safe behavior in the home. Safety in the home can begin with how one does things. The nurse can offer some suggestions for safe behaviors:

- Move slowly and carefully, especially on stairs, when getting accustomed to new glasses, bifocals in particular.
- Avoid loose, floppy slippers without soles. Wear shoes and slippers that fit securely and have nonskid soles and heels.
- Avoid long, flowing, loose clothing, which might cause you to trip.
- Use canes and other assistive devices if you need them.
- Never hold objects in both hands when walking or climbing stairs.

Guidelines for Safety

Floors

- Floors should neither be waxed nor have a high-gloss finish.
- Do not use throw rugs.
- Clutter should be eliminated so pathways will be wide.
- Light cords should not be in pathways.
- Hallways should be well lighted.

Stairways

- Stairways should be well lighted.
- There should be a light switch at the top and bottom of each stairway. It should be a different color than the wall, and it should be a couple of feet ahead of the first step.
- Stairways should have handrails on both sides, if possible, and handrails should extend fully past the top and bottom steps.
- Carpeting should not be loose or torn; no nails should protrude.
- Put colored tape on the edge of both the top and the bottom step.
- The edge of each step should be easy to see. If patterned carpeting makes this difficult, put nonskid strips on the edge of each step.

Bathroom

- Use nonskid mats in the tub, shower, and on the floor (Fig. 7-3).
- Grab bars should be attached to the structural supports in the wall, through the tile.

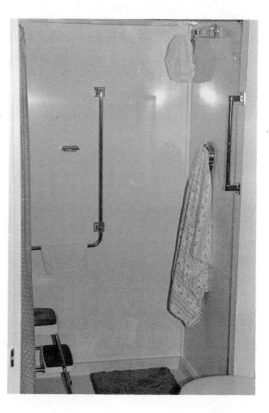

Figure 7–3. A senior-safe shower has grab bars, mat, and a stool to sit on.

- The bathroom should have a night light.
- Keep soap in a dish or get soap on a rope to prevent it from falling where it can cause you to slip.
- Only hold on to grab bars — never towel racks or other wall-attached things (like a soap dish) — when getting in and out of tub, or on and off a stool.
- Never touch electrical appliances when wet or standing on a wet floor.
- Check the temperature of the water before getting into the bathtub to avoid being burned.

Living Room

- The room should have ample lighting, especially near chairs where you sit to read.
- Keep the coffee table close to the couch so you do not trip over it.
- Clear all pathways.
- If you use extension cords, do not use staples to attach them to the walls because you may damage the wires. This is a fire hazard. Don't hide them under carpets, because walking on wires is also damaging.
- Don't overload circuits by having more than two plugs in an electrical outlet.

Bedroom

- The bedside lamp should have a switch on its base or on the cord. The lamp should have a solid base.
- Keep a flashlight next to the bed and check it frequently.
- Periodically check the electric blanket to be sure wires are not coming through and that there are no burned spots. Don't tuck electric blankets under the mattress.
- Do not smoke in bed.
- The path to the bathroom should be clear.
- Use a night light.
- Have the phone next to the bed in easy reach. Keep a list of important phone numbers (police, fire department, and close relative) in large letters near the phone. In fact, keep such a list near each phone.

Kitchen

- Be sure you keep the handles of pans on the stove turned in and away from your pathway.
- Keep flammable, combustible items such as solvents and cleaning fluids away from the stove.
- Keep dishtowels, pot holders and paper towels away from burners.
- Never lean on a burner.
- Do not wear garments with loose-fitting sleeves that can get caught on pan handles or catch fire from burners.
- Close all drawers and cabinet doors.
- It is easy to confuse rows of cans. Separate all insecticides and cleaning fluids from food, and keep out of reach of children.
- Wipe up all spills on floor immediately to avoid slipping.
- Make sure lights on countertops are working and are adequate to avoid injury when working with knives.
- Keep at least 60-watt bulbs in ceiling light fixtures.
- Don't stand on chairs; use step stools.
- When standing on stool to reach something, the object you want should be right in front of you—not off to the side, requiring a long reach.
- Keep a fire extinguisher in the kitchen.
- Keep broilers, ovens, and ducts free of grease to prevent fire.

Fire Hazards in the Home

Besides those fire hazards mentioned in specific situations, there are other fire hazards that the nurse may need to mention:

- Smoking, especially where you might fall asleep
- Improperly used or maintained portable heaters
- Faulty or dirty heating systems and chimneys
- Failure to use fireplace screens
- Overloaded circuits, frayed cords, faulty wiring, and defective appliances
- Accumulations of newspaper, magazines, and rags
- Improperly stored solvents, paint supplies, and liquid fuel

Smoke detectors are imperative—one or several—depending on the size of a home. Guidelines for safety outside the home are discussed in the display below.

Safety Outside the Home

Dos and Don'ts

- Do watch closely for curbs, cracks in the pavement, and objects you could trip over.
- Do consider a railing for outside steps and an outside shelf to hold packages (while you open the door).
- Do plan exit routes from your house or apartment in case of fire. Don't use elevators.
- Do maintain the steps, pavement, and lawn.
- Do have rubber tips put on canes and other walking aids; adaptable ice-gripping ends are also available. Tips should be at least 1½ inches in diameter and should be kept clean. Cane handles can be built up with rubber or cloth covered with tape for a better grip.
- Do have correct change ready for public transport; keep alert and brace yourself for sudden stops and starts.
- Don't rush across the street, especially in bad weather; walk cautiously and look for traffic.
- Don't feel embarrassed about asking someone for a seat on public transportation. Often they don't offer for fear help won't be well received. It is safer to sit than to stand.
- Don't be overvigorous with exercise, especially new tasks such as snow shoveling.
- Don't use separate door latches and locks; one strong [dead bolt] lock is adequate and is easily opened (allows easy exit in case of fire.)

(Courtesy of Brown County Commission on Aging, Green Bay, Wisconsin)

Driving a Car

Driving a car may be an older person's most cherished symbol of independence. Two safety messages, other than general safe driving habits, are important for older drivers. The nurse can make these important suggestions:

- Do not drive when you have taken medication that can slow reaction time or cause drowsiness.
- Observe both maximum and minimum speed limits. Driving too *slowly* can be as dangerous as exceeding the maximum speed limit.

Safe Use of Medications

From statistics gathered by the National Council on Patient Information and Education, it is apparent that medication misuse by elderly people is a serious problem. About 40% of those who suffer adverse drug reactions are over age 60. One sixth of the people over age 70 who are admitted to the hospital have a problem related to a drug reaction. One out of four nursing home admissions is the result of an inability to take medications correctly. Many of the elderly save drugs because they are "too expensive to throw away," they share drugs with friends if they have some of the same health problems, and they mix pills up by putting them all in the same bottle. The nurse can provide instructions that foster safety in the use of medications:

- Go through your medicine cabinet every six months and throw out medications that do not have labels, that you no longer take, or that are outdated.
- Use a color-coded calendar or chart and pill holders to keep track of pills for days and times they should be taken. Drugstores sell many kinds of pill boxes. Your doctor, nurse, or pharmacist will help you make the chart or calendar.
- If you cannot read a label, ask the pharmacist to make one with larger type.
- Do not take anyone else's medications or share yours.
- Be sure your doctor knows all the over-the-counter medicines you are taking.
- Check with your doctor regularly to see if you still need all your medications.
- Be sure you understand how to take all the medicines you buy over the counter.
- For every prescription you get, also get clear instructions on by what route to take it, how much to take and when, how long to take it, what it is for, side effects to watch for, and what food or medicine you cannot take with it (Fig. 7-4).
- Ask about generic prescriptions.
- Carry a list in your purse or wallet of all the drugs you are taking.

First Aid Measures for Independent Living

An older person living alone must be prepared for emergencies. A First Aid kit is essential. Four common medical emergencies are heart attacks, choking, trauma, and burns.

Offer the older person some basic instructions for first aid:

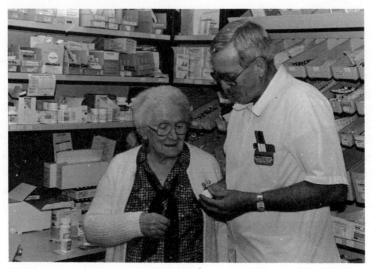

Figure 7–4. *For every prescription, get clear instructions on what, why, how, and when to take it and what to watch for.*

- In case of any unusual chest pain or shortness of breath, dial your emergency phone number or a rescue squad; then relax as comfortably as you can, loosen clothing, and do not eat or drink.
- If you choke on a piece of food, try a forceful cough. If that does not dislodge the chunk of food, try to reach it with your finger. Gagging or vomiting may bring it out. Otherwise get to a countertop or another solid piece of furniture and reach across it to grab the other side. Quickly and firmly, press your lower chest and upper abdomen against the edge. Use the *side* and not a corner. This should work if you do it hard enough.
- Run *only* cold water or apply *only* cold wet cloths to a burn while you wait for help.
- If you suspect a broken bone, try to call for help and then rest the limb up on a pillow until help arrives.
- Put direct pressure with a towel or other clean cloth on a cut that is bleeding and hold the wound at heart level or higher if you can.

Protection Against Crime

Crimes against elderly people range from fraud to physical abuse. Local police departments are a source of information on how the elderly can protect themselves from all kinds of crime (see Chap. 1).

Mental and Emotional Wellness

Stress

Stress is a state of tension, of body or mind, that acts on the nervous system. Responses of the nervous system include relaxation of the bronchial tubes, constriction of blood vessels in the stomach and intestines, and the pumping of more blood from the heart to the skeletal muscles. There is increased release of glucose from the liver, increased activity of the sweat glands, and the production of more adrenalin.

Common stressors are pain or unpleasant excitement such as fear, anger, or insecurity. When stress is caused by a real emergency, such as impending danger, the person will have a pounding heart, rapid breathing, and "goose pimples," and feel as if every hair is standing on end. This condition, when the body is ready for some kind of action, is called a "fight or flight" response.

A certain amount of stress is desirable, as it motivates one toward learning, activity, and growth. Too much stress diminishes one's ability to cope and has negative results. Excessive response to stress may predispose one to disorders and disease, a few of which are headaches, hypertension, peptic ulcers, and colitis.

Stressors in Older People

Some stressors in psychosocial adjustments to aging are very traumatic, such as loss of health and loss of significant others (see Chap. 5). Role transitions may be accompanied by conflict and mixed feelings. For example, one may be very happy to retire before age 65 until others begin to say things like, "You're too *young* to retire," or "What will you do with all your time?" Then feelings of guilt may develop. Regret at giving up a role where one has felt useful is a common feeling even when the prospect of retirement is pleasing. There may be a loss of power in the role transition from worker to retiree that diminishes self-esteem.

A significant factor is that in old age, stress situations can occur so closely in time that attempts to cope are unsuccessful. Grief can remain unresolved if one loss is followed quickly by another, like the death of a loved one, the development of a health problem, and a change in the environment. Life can be experienced as a constant state of fear, anger, and insecurity. The older person cannot physiologically recover from prolonged stress as fast as the younger person recovers. Illness is a common outcome.

Signs of Stress

Numerous physical signs of stress in the older person are similar to aging changes. Among them are elevated blood pressure, urinary frequency, diarrhea, increased heart rate, dyspnea, insomnia, and fatigue. Following are some of the mental and emotional signs of stress:

- Lack of attention to details
- Lack of concentration
- Lack of interest
- Lack of awareness to external stimuli
- Living in the past
- Forgetfulness
- Tearfulness
- Withdrawal
- Paranoia
- Depression
- Irritability
- Feelings of worthlessness

Management of Stress: Nursing Implications

Stress is a normal part of life, so stress management is a lifelong effort. It is helpful if one can maintain a healthy life-style and keep the stresses of life in perspective. Suggestions on how to do this can be offered to the older person:

- Accept responsibility for your own life, happiness, and well-being
- Set realistic goals
- Solve problems one step at a time
- Know when you need help and ask for it
- Try to be flexible and keep a positive attitude
- Stay healthy and physically active
- Take time to "smell the roses"

The nurse's role in stress management is mainly to provide education. The older person can be instructed in self-help for managing stress in wellness classes, and in one-on-one situations. An example of the latter is when a nurse takes an older person's blood pressure and talks with him about it. She might ask, "Does your blood pressure go up if you get tense or upset?" If the answer is yes, then she might say, "Deep breathing is a good way to help keep your blood pressure down at a time like that." An explanation of what is meant by deep breathing should follow (see "Guidelines for Relaxation").

Role of Exercise

Appropriate and regular exercise increases mental health and is effective in relieving tensions caused by stress. Yoga for beginners is excellent for older people because it is slow-paced. Instruction incorporates deep breathing, relaxation, and reflection on one's inner self. There is a wealth of information about yoga available on audio and videotape cassettes and in books. As with all exercise, the older person chooses what feels com..ortable. The cross-legged position so often pictured with yoga need not discourage the older person. Many yoga movements can be done when one is lying or sitting. One will find, however, that gradually working into yoga and trying different positions, even if they must be modified, will be rewarding. Flexibility and joint mobility will be improved, and this feeling of accomplishment helps lift the spirits and contribute to positive thinking. Throughout yoga instructions there are suggestions for mental relaxation.

Guidelines for Relaxation

The nurse can instruct the older adult in ways to call on inner resources for meditating, positive thinking, and relaxation:

1. In meditation, the focus on proper breathing clears the mind. Sit in a quiet place with your spine straight and close your eyes. Release all thoughts from your mind. Take a deep breath; fill and expand the chest and abdomen. Hold it, silently count to three, and exhale completely. Repeat twice. Then continue with the deep breathing but concentrate on the flow of your breath in and out of your nostrils. This will keep your mind empty of the everyday clutter and make you feel peaceful. Now picture the most quiet, pleasant place you have ever been, and imagine that you are there now. Stay there as long as you wish.
2. Begin with the breathing as described in step 1. Then when you have established a restful breathing pattern, start with your toes and concentrate on relaxing muscles in each part of your body.
3. Begin the same as in step 2, establishing a breathing pattern. When you feel calm, repeat one of these affirmations a number of times:
   "I have within me everything I need to help myself."
   "I love and am loved."
   "The more I give, the more I receive."
   "Only positive things affect me."

Another relaxation technique is to lie down and, after a minute or two of deep breathing, concentrate on the thought that with each exhalation you are growing lighter and lighter, finally floating away.

Working at a Job

More and more older people are retiring from jobs and then discovering that they want new ones. As part of the Worker Equity Initiative, the American Association of Retired Persons has developed a series of career-development and job-search workshops designed to assist the older worker in efforts to find suitable employment. The nurse can suggest this resource and also tell the older person that there are books on career counseling specifically for people his age. Job placement for people over age 50 is a service that may be offered by community organizations in large cities. For some people, the work force is the only place for them to feel useful. Whether or not an older person is actually looking for employment may not be what matters — knowing he has value in the job market is a boost to his ego.

The intergenerational benefits of working is the opportunity for older and younger workers to get to know and appreciate one another. The mind of the older person is stimulated by contact with other age groups and the sharing of ideas and opinions.

Rewards of Volunteerism

It is never too late to volunteer, and one is never too old to be useful. Hospitals offer many opportunities for the older person who wants to get involved in volunteer work. There is a never-ending need for volunteers to do tasks such as stuffing envelopes for large mailings or delivering mail or flowers. The primary reward is to hear someone say, "We don't know what we'd do without you." An older person with culinary skills can become invaluable to the dietary department. Spending one morning every week cutting vegetables and fruits to prepare the salad bar in the cafeteria can be extremely satisfying.

Belonging to organizations is another way to volunteer. Working in church clubs and on committees helps older persons to stay in touch with their peers.

The beauty of volunteering is that one is in control of one's time, even when on a schedule. This control reinforces the feeling of independence. Days and hours are negotiable and the volunteer is always appreciated.

Learning and Growing

Older persons have numerous opportunities to learn everything for self-development from crafts to history. Health and wellness classes and screening programs like those for diabetes and high blood pressure are geared to self-care. Any idea can be adapted in some way to small group activities or used in wellness promotion by the nurse.

Community resources or sponsoring organizations include universities, colleges, libraries, the YMCA, the YWCA, churches, hospitals, and agencies on aging. A chamber of commerce or a large shopping mall may sponsor a health fair. Financial service organizations offer workshops in controlling money. Banks are becoming more involved with their growing numbers of older clients. Their clubs for people over 50, 55, 60, or 65 may sponsor monthly social and learning activities and offer "house calls" and financial counseling (Fig. 7-5).

Self-development classes and programs include foreign languages, music and art appreciation, basic acting, creative writing, starting your own business, personality development, astrology, religion, genealogy, and using computers.

Newspapers and magazines frequently report that middle-aged people are becoming more and more interested in their own health. Nurses can offer classes on staying healthy, which should be open to people age 50

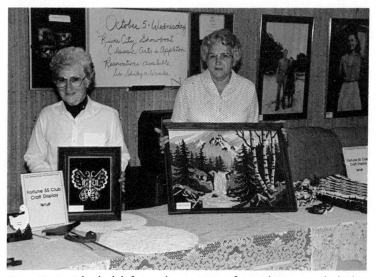

Figure 7–5. A bank club for people over 55 is a financial resource, which also offers social activities and opportunities to learn and sell crafts.

and older. Such classes should focus on normal functions, prevention of disease, and information on common problems:

Stress Prevention
How the Body Functions (one system at a time)
Cancer Detection
Do You Have Diabetes?
Risk Factors in Heart Disease
Preventing Infections
Coping With Grief
Preventing Heat Stroke

Rights under Medicare and the "mysteries" of Medicare, in general, should be discussed on an ongoing basis. Older people need regular opportunities to seek answers to questions about their health.

Sexuality

Maintaining one's sexuality — growing as a desirable male or female — is an important aspect of wellness at any age. The normal aging process does not preclude sexual activity. Impotence in men and lack of sexual response in women are not natural results of growing older. Many women report an increase in sexual desire once the years of childbearing are over and menopause has passed. In both men and women, the desire and need to participate in sexual activity can remain strong throughout a lifetime. With age and experience, sex can be extremely satisfying.

Aging Changes and Sexual Response

Dryness of the vaginal walls, making penetration difficult, is the only aging change that directly affects sexual intercourse. This can be remedied by application of a water-soluble gel. For women, orgasms may be less intense than those experienced at a younger age but just as pleasurable. The clitoris remains highly sensitive to stimulation. Other physiological responses to sexual intimacy, such as flushed skin and breast enlargement, may diminish, but these diminished responses do not interfere with pleasure.

As a man ages, his ability to initiate an erection usually declines. However, he may be able to maintain it longer. There is less urgency to ejaculate, which may bring more enjoyment to the sexual act because it can be prolonged. The emphasis in coitus for older people is on quality rather than quantity. For men, especially, this may be hard to accept because they tend to equate manhood with the ability to have frequent sexual intercourse. Expressions of tenderness, including touching, hugging, and kissing, or just being close to a significant other, may be more satisfying to an older person than sexual intercourse.

Societal Attitudes

To a large extent, the sexual freedom in today's society has not been extended to older people. Sex is not generally considered normal and healthy in later life. The association of aging with disease, weakness, and frailty has contributed to the notion that sex in old age is unnecessary, unlikely, or impossible. It is common in all age groups, even among the elderly, to regard sex as inappropriate for older people. In a society where sex appeal and sexual ability have been linked to youthful beauty this is understandable. The labels "dirty old man" or "dirty old woman" may be applied in good humor, but they are often the result of ignorance and of perceptions based on negative images of aging. Sensitive to the attitudes of others, many older persons feel foolish or guilty about their need for and enjoyment of sexual activities.

Psychological Barriers

History of Sexual Image

Today's elderly women were raised during a period when sex was considered appropriate only in marriage and, for many women, only for the purpose of procreation. They were victims of silence on the subject of anatomy and sexual functioning. Wives performed their "duty" in the marriage bed, and enjoyment of sex was a revelation that many of them felt was not quite proper. An elderly man would probably admit that he was encouraged to "sow his wild oats" by having sex with "bad girls" before he married a "good" one.

Traditional sexual roles required men to be aggressive and women to be submissive. This must have been inhibiting for the woman with strong sexual desires, and demoralizing for the man who was growing older. Thus, many married people reach old age with a fair share of problems related to sexuality that have little to do with age. People in their 50s and 60s are the children of these marriages. They are familiar with these attitudes and have adopted some of them.

Another psychological barrier to sexual activity that stems from the history of the older population is that masturbation is sinful, harmful, or both. In reality, masturbation, mutual or solitary, can be beneficial in releasing sexual tensions.

Fear of Illness or Injury

A common fear among older people is that sexual intercourse may cause a heart attack. While sexual activity does require exertion, a heart attack is not likely. For those people who have a history of coronary disease, instruction on the signs of stress is necessary. These include dizziness, shortness of breath, rapid, pounding heart rate, and diaphoresis. Any of these would necessitate halting sexual activity until medical advice can be obtained.

An older person who has had surgery on the hip or back is frequently afraid of reinjuring the operated area or causing a complication. Clear postoperative instructions on what movements to avoid at *all* times will be guidelines for sexual practices. For a person with arthritis, no position is harmful if it does not cause discomfort. Arthritis medication and warm baths or applications to the joints prior to sexual activity will benefit these people.

Medications

A number of drugs used in the treatment of coronary disease, hypertension, and chronic depression can cause sexual dysfunction. This fact underlines the importance of teaching older patients about the medications they are taking and urging them to consult their physician when problems arise.

Loss of a Partner

Death of a spouse or loved one is a sad fact of old age. Divorce is not uncommon. For the single elderly person, establishing a sexual relationship may cause moral dilemmas. Women may experience guilt and anxiety at the thought of sex without marriage. An elderly man may find the role of suitor difficult if he feels he is becoming sexually inadequate. Years of making love to the same partner — perhaps the first and only — may make one timid about becoming intimate with someone new when the body one has to share is sagging and wrinkled. In all cases, seeking new sexual relationships in later years means readjustment and risk. The older person may not feel it is worth the effort.

Nursing Implications

An active sex life is healthy. In old age, a person with a positive self-image, a background of loving relationships, and opportunities for satisfactory sexual expression is more likely to maintain sexual wellness. Some people go through life uncomfortable with and negative about the whole idea of sex. Sexuality is a personal matter. When there are concerns, a person might be reluctant to discuss them. The nurse cannot be certain about a person's attitudes and self-image. Wellness promotion in this sensitive area demands tact.

Here are some ways to teach and promote sexual health:

- Show respect for an older person by addressing him according to his wishes.
- Acknowledge and reinforce sexual identity and pride by commenting on an older person's attractiveness as a male or female when appropriate. For example: "You have a good barber, Mr. M," or "Mrs. J, the color of your dress makes your cheeks pink."
- Stress the effect of general good health on sexuality.
- Encourage moderation in food and drink. Too much food or alcohol diminishes sexual desire and ability.
- Check the older person's knowledge of side effects of drugs and give needed instruction as to their effect on sexual ability.
- Appropriately refer older persons for medical counseling about hormone replacement, penile prostheses, and other aids to sexual activity. There are a number available.
- In all wellness promotion settings, try to have written information available on sexuality because many older persons hesitate to ask questions about it.

Dealing with Chronic Discomfort

Chronic discomfort due to disease is common in old age and must be considered in a discussion of wellness. Pain intrudes on one's life-style by imposing restrictions on activity and by requiring one to change existing habits. Although pain is depressing and treatment can be expensive, proper self-care and a good support system can allow the older person with chronic pain to achieve and maintain a level of wellness that permits him to function independently. There is no doubt that a positive outlook, good humor, and laughter help alleviate all kinds of pain. Stress management techniques also can be beneficial in pain control. Older persons need to be made aware of these facts. There are practical ways to help the older person live with chronic pain (Table 7-2).

Table 7-2. *Helping Older People Live with Discomforts of Common Chronic Conditions*

Disease/Condition	Discomfort	Teach Older Person/Family the Following:

I. Cardiovascular problems (lack of oxygen to myocardium)	Chest pain	a. Understand what is happening in the heart when the problem occurs (to reduce anxiety).
		 b. Recognize difference between angina attacks and a beginning infarct:
		   1. *Angina.* Pain is intense but *usually* goes away in a few minutes—often described as "indigestion"; may be precipitated by exercise or exertion; relieved by rest and nitroglycerine; pain may spread to shoulder, arm, neck and jaw.
		   2. *Beginning Infarct.* Pain is sudden, severe, sharp; may radiate to left arm and shoulder; comes without exertion, lasts longer, and is *not* relieved with rest and nitroglycerine.
		 c. Understand use of nitrates.
		 d. Choose activities to save energy.
		 e. Understand early signs of fatigue.

II. Peripheral vascular disease (arterial occlusion or arteriosclerosis of lower extremities)	Leg pain and limping (claudication)	a. Avoid injury to legs. b. Plan rest periods for elevating legs. c. Wear elastic stockings. d. Avoid circular garters. e. Plan daily chores to eliminate unnecessary walking. f. Walk regularly to build up tolerance. g. Don't sit with legs crossed. h. Seek physician's advice on analgesics.

III. Peptic or stomach ulcer (open sore in mucous lining) Hiatal hernia (protrusion of stomach into chest through an opening in diaphragm)	Epigastric discomfort	a. Understand and use antacids properly. b. Eat those foods in those amounts that minimize pain. c. If lying flat in bed aggravates the problem, sleep on several pillows. d. Avoid physical activity that contributes to the problem.
IV. Osteoporosis (progressive loss of bone mass, causing weaker bone)	Back pain	a. Sit and stand erect. Good posture relieves strain on spine and back muscles. b. Exercise to keep abdominal muscles strong to help support spine. c. Maintain ideal weight. d. Ask physician about back supports.
V. Rheumatoid arthritis (a systemic disease with joint inflammation, swelling, and destruction, characterized by acute attacks and remissions)	Joint pain (joints may be extra stiff in morning on arising)	a. Exercise range of motion regularly within limits of pain to prevent contractures. b. Get extra rest. c. Avoid positions of prolonged flexion of involved joints to prevent contractures. d. Use splints for hands as necessary, at night (physician's prescription required). e. Take medication faithfully. f. Use warm baths, packs, on painful joints. Check with physician about paraffin baths.
VI. Osteoarthritis (mechanical wearing of joints; degenerative joint disease, or DJD)	Joint pain (at night or following weightbearing)	a. Reduce stress on joints by avoiding long periods of standing or walking. b. Practice good posture. c. Keep weight down. d. Stay mobile.

Teaching an older person how to live with the effects of chronic disease promotes wellness. A teaching program is based on how the individual is able to carry out activities of daily living, interact with others, work at home or at a job, and participate in leisure activities (see Chap. 8 for discussion of common chronic diseases).

Promoting Spiritual Wellness

One cannot define another person's spiritual wellness, but there are some general characteristics:

- Acceptance of one's right to feel whole
- Belief in a purpose for one's own life
- Absence of fear
- The capacity for loving and accepting love in return
- A sense of oneness with and responsibility for all other human beings
- A sense of being one with the planet and the universe

If one believes in spiritual wellness then one must believe that there are resources that are helpful in achieving it, such as a personal concept of God or the universe, and religious or spiritual beliefs. Older persons who talk to nurses about God, religion, spirituality, and reasons for being may need to verbalize concerns or find answers to questions that will help them to live peacefully. The nurse is best equipped to assist older persons in this kind of soul searching if she has reflected on a personal definition of spiritual wellness and has basic knowledge of a wide spectrum of religious and spiritual beliefs.

Summary

Wellness is a continuous process of maintaining harmony between a total person and his environment. Each person has his own definition of wellness, and the nurse must work with this in mind. Self-care is part of good health. The changes brought about by the aging process make staying well a challenge. Older persons need emotional support and health education in order to help themselves stay well.

Exercise is a major factor in wellness, and it can be incorporated into the life-style of any person. A diet based on the four basic food groups is essential, although problems of aging, loneliness, and reduced income may discourage older persons from eating well. Older persons must be taught to take care of their bodies.

A safe environment is a consideration in wellness and involves taking medications properly, keeping the home free of hazards that cause accidents, knowing how to maneuver in public, and knowing how to avoid being a victim of crime. An older person should know what to do in case of medical emergency.

Learning to manage stress keeps one healthy. Sexuality is natural at any age, and the sexual aspect of an older person must be recognized. The nurse must remember that keeping busy and useful is part of each person's wellness, and she must be aware of opportunities for older persons to do so. Chronic pain often accompanies health problems of old age, so older persons should be instructed in how to live with their discomfort, what to expect of pain, and how to recognize when pain may be a sign that something is wrong.

Activities

1. Ask a well older person for advice on how to maintain wellness while aging.
2. Choose one of the following activities for sharing in class:
   a. Investigate locations of senior fitness programs in your town. What is the age range of those who participate? Describe the activities.
   b. Visit a supermarket. Read some labels, and compare prices. Write some specific suggestions for wise shopping for an older couple on a limited budget who should follow low-fat, low-carbohydrate diets.
   c. Investigate restaurants and make a list of those that accommodate the diets and budgets of older persons. Discuss the ways they meet their particular requirements.
3. What steps would you have to take to make your home or apartment safe for seniors?
4. Make a wellness poster that would be appropriate for a senior center.
5. How would you answer these questions asked by older people?
   a. "I have arthritis in my shoulders. How can I exercise?"
   b. "What vitamins should I take? I already take Vitamin E and B and calcium."
   c. "My mother died of a stroke at 66. I'm 70. What can I do so that doesn't happen to me?"
6. Write a week of menus for a healthy 70-year-old woman who weighs 170 pounds and is 5'7" tall.
7. Make four general suggestions for total wellness.

Bibliography

Benison B, Hogstel M: Aging and movement therapy: essential interventions for the immobile elderly. J Gerontol Nurs 12:8–16, 1986

Bowers A, Thompson J: Clinical Manual of Health Assessment. St. Louis, CV Mosby, 1984

Burggraf V, Donlon B: Assessing the elderly, Part 1: System by system. Am J Nurs 85:974–984, 1985

Burnside I: Nursing and the Aged: A Self-Care Approach, 3rd ed. New York, McGraw-Hill, 1988

Butler R: Don't take it easy—exercise! Nurs Homes 32:34–35, 1983

Dudek S: Nutrition Handbook for Nursing Practice. Philadelphia, JB Lippincott, 1987

Ebersole P, Hess P: Toward Healthy Aging: Human Needs and Nursing Response, 2nd ed. St. Louis, CV Mosby, 1985

Kreulter P: Nutrition in Perspective. Englewood Cliffs, Prentice-Hall, 1980

Lamb K, Miller J, Hernandez M, et al: Falls in the elderly: causes and prevention. Orthop Nurs 6:45–49, 1987

Lampman R: Evaluating and prescribing exercise for elderly patients. Geriatrics 42:63–76, 1987

Lewis M: Sexual activity in later life: a challenging issue for nurses. Imprint 31:48–49, 1984

Merry J: Take your assessment all the way down to the toes. RN 51:60–63, 1988

Olivo J: Developing an exercise program for the elderly with osteoarthritis. Orthop Nurs 6:23–26, 1987

Parsons M, Levy J: Nursing process in injury prevention. J Gerontol Nurs 13:36–40, 1987

Patrick G, Mason L: Special pull-out self-help guide. Part I: How to protect yourself from crime. Part II: First aid when you're alone. Senior Scene. Fall, 19–23, 1987

Raab D, Raab M: Nutrition and aging: an overview. Can Nurs 81:24–26, 1985

Spradley B: Community Health Nursing: Concepts and Practice, 2nd ed. Boston, Little Brown and Co, 1985

Stanton A: Care of the elderly: happy birthday . . . screening the well elderly and their carers. Comm Outlook, Mar. 20–21, 1987

Suitor C, Crowley M: Nutrition Principles and Application in Health Promotion. Philadelphia, JB Lippincott, 1984

Sullivan J, Deane D: Humor and health (CEU exam questions). J Gerontol Nurs 14:20–42, 1988

Yurick A, Spier B, Robb S et al: The Aged Person and the Nursing Process, 2nd ed. New York, Appleton-Century-Crofts, 1984

8

Common Diseases and Disorders of the Aging Person

Learning Objectives

When you complete this chapter, you should be able to:

1. Give examples of the following for cardiovascular disease:
   a. Types
   b. Symptoms
   c. Treatment
   d. Risk factors
2. Discuss respiratory problems and their prognoses in older people.
3. Describe general symptoms of gastrointestinal disease and disorders in older people.
4. List contributing factors in constipation.
5. Give the reasons for symptoms of renal failure.
6. List the most common genitourinary problems in aging people with the treatment for each.
7. Differentiate between multiple myeloma, rheumatoid arthritis, osteoarthritis, osteoporosis and Paget's disease.
8. Define TIA, CVA, and Parkinson's disease.
9. List the signs of a stroke.
10. Identify factors that interfere with the diagnosis and treatment of diabetes in the elderly.
11. Explain the development and treatment of decubitus ulcers.
12. Compare and contrast the common mental disorders of older people.
13. Discuss the differences in cancer treatment and prevention in older people as compared to younger people.

A close relationship exists between age-related changes and diseases in older people. Normal physical problems can be mistaken for signs and symptoms of disease. On the other hand, disease goes undiagnosed when aches and pains are written off as signs of aging. There is a story about a very old man who went to his doctor with a painful right knee, only to have the doctor tell him that he was "just getting old."

"I don't know, doc," the man replied, shaking his head, "my left knee is the same age and it doesn't hurt at all."

In this chapter, the more common diseases and disorders of old age will be briefly described along with the treatment. Medical–surgical textbooks can provide in-depth information. The nurse is concerned with the patient's responses to disease, and her nursing care plan centers on solving and preventing problems related to many factors other than the disease (see Chap. 9).

Cardiovascular Disease

Cardiovascular disease is common in the elderly. Age-related changes and life-style are contributing factors. One heart condition can be a risk factor in causing another. For example, recurrent myocardial ischemia can lead to congestive heart failure.

Coronary Artery Disease

Arteriosclerosis is a thickening and hardening of the arterial walls. Atherosclerosis, in which plaque accumulates on the walls of the arteries, is a form of arteriosclerosis. Narrowing of the arteries caused by this condition results in a reduced supply of blood to the heart upon exertion. If the heart muscle does not get blood, it does not get oxygen, and chest pain or angina pectoris occurs. (The term *angina pectoris* is usually shortened to "angina" in most references.) Repeated or prolonged loss of the oxygen supply to the heart muscles, myocardial ischemia, causes death of the tissue or myocardial infarction.

In the older person, pain may be mild or absent. When pain is reported, the person can often relate it to a particular activity, such as eating a large meal. Instead of pain, the older person may experience a feeling of heaviness under the sternum, shortness of breath, and indigestion. With an angina attack the pulse may increase; the blood pressure can either rise or fall. The skin may be cool, clammy, and pale. Symptoms may be masked by decreased feelings of pain or by memory deficits, and the disease advances undetected.

The treatment involves educating the patient about activities that must be modified to prevent exertion. Patients should also be advised to avoid emotional stress and overeating. Patients with coronary artery disease should keep their weight down and should not smoke. Nitroglycerine is the usual medication prescribed.

Congestive Heart Failure

The heart fails when it loses its ability to pump blood effectively and congestion occurs in the circulatory system. Failure of the left ventricle produces pulmonary edema. There is accumulation of fluid in the tissues and engorgement of the liver. The jugular vein becomes distended. There is fluid and electrolyte imbalance, less cardiac reserve, and a reduced flow of blood to the skeletal muscles and the brain.

Arteriosclerosis, coronary artery disease, myocardial infarction, hypertension, and any other disease or defect that decreases the efficiency of the heart's pumping action may cause it to fail. Pathologies in other systems, such as the kidneys or liver, can precipitate heart failure. Inappropriate drug therapy, malnutrition, and obesity are contributing causes.

The syndrome (or set of symptoms) that results from congestive heart failure may differ from person to person. Symptoms include the following:

- Shortness of breath and dyspnea on exertion
- Orthopnea, the inability to breathe while lying down
- Paroxysmal nocturnal dyspnea — severe nighttime orthopnea
- Excessive fatigue and weakness
- Persistent cough that may produce blood-tinged sputum
- Wheezing on exertion
- Edema, especially noticeable in fingers, feet, and ankles; feet and ankles most swollen when standing
- Feeling of heaviness in muscles
- Confusion, anxiety
- Nausea, vomiting, anorexia
- Right upper quadrant discomfort

Congestive heart failure can be gradual or acute, and it is often the end-stage of heart disease.

The treatment is to reduce the work load on the heart as much as possible. Teaching the patient to plan activities to avoid exertion is imperative. Weight reduction and dietary sodium restriction are important. Drugs include digitalis, diuretics, and vasodilators. A mild tranquilizer may be helpful.

Hypertension

Hypertension is a consistently elevated blood pressure above normal for a given age. It must be noted that "normal" varies according to different authorities. A systolic blood pressure above 140mm HG and a diastolic pressure above 90mm HG can be called high enough to warrant observation in a healthy older person. However, each elderly person is given individual consideration before a diagnosis of hypertension is made. Hypertension in old age is caused by arteriosclerosis and increased resistance in peripheral blood vessels. Genetics may be a factor. The effects of smoking, alcohol, and diet on blood pressure in older people are not clear.

Older people with hypertension may complain of dizziness, headaches, blurred vision, and nosebleeds. Hypertension is linked to strokes, heart damage, and renal failure. Treatment is weight reduction, if necessary, antihypertensive drugs, and limiting sodium in the diet.

Miscellaneous Heart Problems

Other heart conditions can reduce the efficiency of the heart:

Arrhythmias

An arrhythmia is an irregularity in the heartbeat. Occasional abnormal beats are not unusual in a normal older person. Causes of arrhythmias are digitalis toxicity, potassium depletion, infections, and angina. Arrhythmias are treated by digitalis preparations to slow and strengthen the heartbeat and by potassium supplements.

Valvular Disease

The most common cause of diseased values is rheumatic fever. Shortness of breath and dyspnea are the symptoms, if the problem is severe enough to cause more than a heart murmur.

Bacterial Endocarditis

Infection of the endocardium is most frequently associated with other infections, and it has a high mortality rate. Diagnosis is difficult because the presenting symptoms may be vague, including weakness, pallor, anemia, and fatigue.

Arteriosclerosis Obliterans

Arteriosclerosis obliterans is a condition in which the arteries in the lower extremities become so blocked that the transport of oxygenated blood to the tissues is impaired. Occlusion of the arteries can be acute or chronic. Older men are more at risk than older women. Additional risk factors are a history of coronary artery disease, cerebrovascular disease, diabetes mellitus, and smoking.

Pain is the main symptom. Intermittent claudication, cramping pain that comes with walking, is extremely common. In advanced cases, patients report cold feet, numbness, tingling, burning pain, or loss of sensation. The skin may be pale or mottled. Pedal pulses are often difficult to locate or are absent. Over a period of time, lack of oxygen causes the legs to take on a shiny appearance. Toenails thicken and hair is sparse on the legs and toes. Leg wounds will not heal well, if at all. A gangrenous limb can be the disastrous outcome.

Treatment attempts to improve circulation to slow the progression of the disease. Programmed walking is often helpful; that is, the patient is instructed to walk until pain sets in, rest, and then walk some more. The head of the bed may be raised three to four inches on blocks to improve circulation at night. Preventing trauma to the legs is also important.

Aneurysms

An aneurysm is a dilatation of a blood vessel due to a weakening in the vessel wall. In older people, aneurysms of the abdominal aorta and of major arteries in the lower extremities are caused by arteriosclerosis.

Abdominal aneurysms may be asymptomatic. Pain is a danger signal because it can mean an increase in the size of the aneurysm and impending or actual rupture. When these aneurysms are untreated, the mortality rate is high. Surgical resection can be successful on an otherwise healthy person.

The femoral and popliteal arteries are sites of aneurysms in the leg. An aneurysm can be diagnosed by palpation and it can be resected. Amputation is necessary if the circulation to the lower extremity is lost.

Venous Thrombosis

The incidence of thrombosis, or the development of blood clots, in the enlarged veins in the calf muscles of older patients is high. This is chiefly due to surgical procedures and to immobility. Surgical procedures on the lower extremities, especially, and the use of a tourniquet predispose the limb to clots. Elderly patients with fractures of the pelvis and lower limbs are highly susceptible. Venous stasis from bed rest and pooling of the blood in the pelvis by prolonged sitting positions will cause formation of thrombi.

Symptoms vary. Slight to moderate edema of the involved leg may be the only symptom, while pain, tenderness, and tightness can be minimal or absent. The calf may be warm to the touch. Pain and edema at the inner ankle can be significant signs. Homan's sign, which is pain in the calf when the foot is dorsiflexed, is present in some cases. Diagnosis may be made by Doppler ultrasonic examination. Treatment is bed rest, elevation of the extremity, anticoagulants, and hot wet packs.

Pulmonary Embolism

Pulmonary embolism is a major killer in older people. An embolus, or blood clot, in a vein breaks off and travels to the lungs where it occludes a pulmonary vessel and causes an infarction in the lung.

The symptoms depend on the size of the clot. Chest pain can be severe, moderate or nonexistent. Pain can be in the shoulder. A patient with a large thrombus may complain of sudden intense pain, shortness of breath, and dyspnea, and he may die in a matter of minutes. Other symptoms are cyanosis, tachycardia, and shock. Patients with small thrombi may have symptoms of pneumonia. Many times a patient with very small thrombi will have no complaints other than "not feeling well." This person may be slightly diaphoretic and have a grayish cast to his face.

The danger in not detecting symptoms of smaller clot formation is that larger clots follow. The symptoms are treated with bed rest, oxygen, and analgesics. Intravenous heparin is given to prevent further thrombus formation.

Chronic Obstructive Pulmonary Disease

Chronic Obstructive Pulmonary Disease (COPD) in older people comprises emphysema, chronic bronchitis, and asthma. COPD is resistance to expiratory airflow, that is, resistance to air leaving the lungs.

Emphysema

Emphysema is characterized by progressive changes in the lung tissue. The alveolar sacs become distended and break down, destroying the capillary bed. The loss of elasticity in the alveoli prevents normal expiration. Fibrous tissue replaces much of the capillary bed and interferes with normal exchange of oxygen and carbon dioxide during respiration.

Chronic Bronchitis

Chronic bronchitis is inflammation of the bronchi with excessive mucous secretion and a persistent cough. Smoking and air pollutants are among the factors causing this condition.

Asthma

Asthma is airflow obstruction caused by spasm of the smooth muscle of the bronchial tubes, swelling of the mucous membrane, and thick bronchial secretions. The classic wheezing occurs as the air tries to move out through narrowed bronchi and bronchioles. Causes of asthma include allergy, infection, and emotional stress.

The signs and symptoms of COPD are shortness of breath and cough. The expiration of air is prolonged. In advanced COPD, a "barrel chest" is apparent.

The treatment of COPD involves long-term planning with the patient, family, physician, nurse, and respiratory therapist. Education is aimed at slowing progression of the disease. The patient should be taught to avoid respiratory irritants and respiratory infection. Depending on the patient's status, pulmonary ventilation is improved by a number of measures:

- Bronchodilating drugs
- Humidification of the air in the patient's immediate environment to loosen secretions
- Intermittent positive-pressure breathing
- Breathing exercises
- Chest percussion and postural drainage
- Oxygen therapy
- Adequate rest
- Extra fluids
- A well-balanced diet

Emotional support is a critical part of the treatment.

Pneumonia

Pneumonia is a lung infection that may be bacterial or viral. In older people, bacterial pneumonia is the most common; in fact, it is one of the leading causes of death in people over 65. The risk of pneumonia is increased by COPD, influenza, lung cancer, alcoholism, and general poor health. The incidence of pneumonia is high among the institutionalized elderly.

An older person frequently has symptoms that are not typical of pneumonia, and the diagnosis is easily missed. Anorexia, weakness, confusion, and lethargy may be the only evidence of a problem, and these symptoms are nonspecific. A respiratory rate over 24, in conjunction with some of these symptoms, is significant and should be promptly investigated. The treatment of pneumonia in elderly people is bed rest, antibiotic therapy, oxygen, and forcing fluids.

Gastrointestinal Disease

Esophageal Disorders

With increased age, esophageal motility is altered by degenerative changes in the smooth muscle. Actually, degeneration in the nervous system affects movement along the entire gastrointestinal tract. If the older person has symptoms of change in esophageal contractions, there will be difficulty in swallowing and substernal pressure. Dietary changes and smaller meals may be helpful.

Hiatal Hernia

A hiatal or diaphragmatic hernia is a protrusion of the stomach through an opening in the diaphragm and into the thoracic cage. The protrusion may occur because of degenerative changes. The incidence of hiatal hernia is extremely high in the elderly population. Signs and symptoms vary. Heartburn or sour stomach may be caused by some kinds of food and tends to be most evident when the person is lying down. Treatment is dietary alteration and antacids, and the patient should keep the head elevated on a number of pillows when lying down.

Chronic Atrophic Gastritis

This is an inflammatory stomach condition, the cause of which is unknown. Symptoms are vague and include loss of appetite, belching, nausea, vomiting, a feeling of fullness, and some discomfort. Antispasmodic drugs and a bland diet of small meals may help relieve symptoms.

Ulcers

An ulcer is an open sore. In older people, both gastric and duodenal ulcers are fairly common. They may be caused by stress, drugs, and chronic gastritis. Pain may be less acute than in younger people. The main symptoms are usually decreased appetite, listlessness, weight loss, black, tarry stools (indicating bleeding), and anemia. Conservative treatment consists of antacids and frequent drinks of low-fat or skim milk. Acid-producing substances such as alcohol, caffeine, and spices should be avoided.

Diverticulosis

Diverticulosis is the presence of tiny hernias or sacs in the mucosa of the large bowel. The most frequent site is the sigmoid portion of the left colon. Contributing factors may be constipation, obesity, emotional tension, or any eating habits that cause sustained muscular contractions. Most people are asymptomatic. Pain in the lower abdomen is the most common symptom and is often relieved by defecation. The condition is treated with diet and with management of constipation. Weight reduction is desirable in cases of obesity. Diverticulitis is inflammation and perforation of a diverticulum with pain and cramping and blood in the stool. This condition requires analgesics, rest, restriction of oral intake, intravenous therapy, and antibiotics.

Hemorrhoids

Hemorrhoids are dilated or swollen veins in the anal area. They can be internal, under the mucous membrane, or external and covered by skin. Hemorrhoids result from the pressure of straining to defecate when one is constipated. The symptoms are itching, bleeding, and pain, especially with bowel movements. Surgery is the least likely treatment option because hemorrhoids do recur. Stool softeners and bulk-forming agents will help reduce constipation. Anesthetic, emollient, or cortisone ointments and suppositories relieve itching and discomfort.

Constipation

Patients who are constipated will *not* respond well to treatment or nursing care until this very basic problem receives attention.

The following factors contribute to causing constipation:

- Lack of intestinal motility, with soft stool remaining in the rectum

- Increased absorption of fluid and altered muscle contractions in the intestine that produce hard, dry, stool that is difficult to expel and may become impacted
- Loss of abdominal muscle tone
- Neglecting the urge to defecate
- Poor dentition that makes it difficult to eat high-fiber food
- Bad eating habits and poor fluid intake
- Chronic use of enemas or laxatives
- Environmental factors such as lack of privacy and changes or disruptions in routines
- Degenerative changes in the nervous system
- The vicious cycle of anal lesions (hemorrhoids and fissures) being caused by and then causing further constipation
- Mental stress or disorder
- Drugs

Renal Failure

Age-related deterioration of the kidneys puts older persons at high risk for renal failure. Diabetes mellitus is a major cause of renal failure since it causes vascular changes in the glomeruli. Other causes of renal failure are chronic kidney disease and urinary tract infections, and long-standing, uncontrolled hypertension. The following are the symptoms, which are due to buildup of metabolic waste products:

- Edema
- Changes in urinary output
- Fatigue and general slowdown
- Memory problems
- Nausea, vomiting, anorexia, and weight loss
- Changes in sleep patterns
- Headaches
- Slurred speech
- Decreased sexual performance and desire
- Dry skin and itching
- Sensations of coldness
- Hypothermia
- Restlessness
- Hiccoughs
- Abnormal muscle movements; jerks, cramps, tremors, gait problems
- Paranoid personality changes
- Impaired vision and hearing

If progression of the disease is slow enough, the body adapts somewhat to the changes in its biochemistry. Acute disease produces the more severe symptoms, and convulsions, coma, and death are a frequent outcome.

Short-term, conservative treatment consists of a low-protein, low-sodium, low-potassium diet and fluid restriction. When the disease advances, dialysis is the next step.

Gallbladder Disease

Gallstones, composed chiefly of calcium and cholesterol, are common in old age, especially in women. Pain is the main symptom. Gallstones can be responsible for obstruction, infection, and inflammation of the gallbladder. Surgical treatment may be required.

Genitourinary Problems

Incontinence

Urinary incontinence is the involuntary escape of urine from the bladder to such a degree that it causes mental and physical distress and curtails social activities. Incontinence is a symptom of numerous other conditions related to the filling and emptying of the bladder. Possible causes of incontinence are infections, obstructions, conditions that affect reflexes and muscle tone, and sphincter weakness. Nervous system disorders can cause incontinence.

Drugs are largely ineffective in treatment. Stress incontinence in women may be relieved by surgery. Urinary incontinence may be managed by appliances that catch the urine and by indwelling catheters. Catheters are not desirable. Clean intermittent catheterization may be tried for atonic bladders.

Drug therapy accounts for some incontinence. Older people may be incontinent simply because physical and environmental conditions may be such that they can not maneuver fast enough to get to a bathroom on time. These problems of incontinence are more easily solved.

Urinary Tract Infections

Infections of the lower urinary tract are very common, and a major cause of fever in the elderly. Risk factors are urinary stasis, poor hygiene, catheters, decreased intake of fluids, immobility, cross infection in institutional settings, and sexual activity. Signs and symptoms may be absent or nonspecific, such as vomiting and fever. Classic symptoms are abdominal discomfort, voiding irregularities, and foul-smelling urine. Treatment is drug therapy, dictated by urine culture results, and increased intake of fluids.

Benign Prostatic Hypertrophy

Enlargement of the prostate gland causes symptoms only when the overgrowth compresses the urethra and causes urinary frequency, hematuria, nocturia, dribbling, hesitancy, retention, or interruption of the stream. Transurethral resection (TUR) to remove the obstructing part of the gland is the most desirable treatment because it does not require an abdominal incision, and a normal postoperative recovery is rapid.

Gynecological Conditions

Age-related changes and muscle damage from childbirth weaken perineal structures and allow herniation of the bladder (cystocele) and rectum (rectocele) into the vagina. A prolapsed uterus is another herniation. The condition is accompanied by lower back pain, incontinence or retention of urine, and constipation. Surgical repair is the best solution.

Senile vaginitis, due to age-related changes in the vaginal wall and secretions is an aggravating condition causing itching, burning, and discharge. Estrogen suppositories and ointments are easy to use and effective.

Musculoskeletal Disorders

Osteoarthritis

Osteoarthritis is often called degenerative joint disease (DJD). In this disease, the joint cartilage and the underlying bone deteriorate. As a result, there is an abnormal growth of bone in and around the joint. Osteoarthritis can be secondary to trauma, old fractures, infection, and neurological, circulatory, and metabolic disorders, and the cause is often unknown. The hip, knee, fingers, and spinal column are commonly affected.

In the hip and the knee, pain that increases with weight-bearing is the main symptom. Stiffness after inactivity and grating noises when walking or bending the knee are also common. The patient with vertebral involvement has backache and symptoms of nerve compression. Osteoarthritis in the fingers is characterized by knobby, frequently painless joints, called Heberden's nodes.

Osteoarthritis is treated by drug therapy to reduce pain and by physical therapy. Joint replacement is done for hips and knees when the condition is intolerable.

Rheumatoid Arthritis

Rheumatoid arthritis is a disease that usually affects younger people. The affected joints are painful, swollen, stiff, red, and warm to the touch. Systemic symptoms of the disease are fatigue, malaise, weakness, weight loss, anorexia, fever, anemia, and wasting. Eventually body organs may be affected by the inflammatory process. Rheumatoid arthritis is more common in women and affects all individuals differently, coming and going throughout a lifetime. Acute attacks of the disease are often related to stress. By old age, the individual has multiple joint and systemic problems. The cause is unknown, but the disease tends to occur in families.

The treatment program involves medication to treat inflammation, rest, adequate nutrition, physical and occupational therapy, and education. The goals are avoiding and reducing pain, preventing deformities, and maintaining good general health.

Paget's Disease

Paget's disease, osteitis deformans, is a slowly progressive condition in which bone is formed in a disorganized pattern. Although the bones become larger, broader, thicker, and heavier, the disorganization of cells makes bones weaker. The most frequently involved bones are the skull, pelvis, spine, femur, and tibia. Paget's disease is almost always seen in people past middle age and more often in men. The cause is unknown.

A person with Paget's disease may be stooped and have bowed legs, large feet, a large head, and a wide pelvis. Spinal nerve compression can cause symptoms. Pain relief and prevention of fractures are treatment priorities. Drugs may be given to reduce bone formation.

Osteoporosis

Osteoporosis is the reduction of bone mass with demineralization. It is more common in older women, and the chief symptom is back pain (see Chap. 7).

Multiple Myeloma

Multiple myeloma is a highly malignant and incurable plasma cell abnormality originating in the bone marrow. Bone destruction by plasma cells occurs in the ribs, sternum, skull, vertebrae, and proximal ends of the long bones. Middle-aged and elderly people are most often affected. The disease is slow, with steadily increasing pain similar to that of arthritis, especially in the back. Calcium accumulating in the bloodstream causes anorexia, nausea and vomiting, constipation, lethargy, confusion, and heart muscle irritability. Abnormal proteins filtering out of the urine cause impaired renal function. Since normal functioning of the plasma cells has to do with immunity, the multiple myeloma patient may have signs of infection.

Fractures

The most common fractures in older people are of the hip, wrist, and humerus. Falls are the usual cause. Compression back fractures in osteoporosis and multiple myeloma must also be mentioned. Symptoms of fractures depend on the type and location of the broken bone. For example, a fracture of the upper humerus affects shoulder joint movement. The extent of muscle damage determines the amount of swelling, bruising, and pain. The treatment of fractures in the older patient depends on the type and location of the broken bone, as well as the overall condition and mobility of the patient. Fractures must be reduced; that is, the bone fragments must be realigned and immobilized until they heal and function can be restored. This is accomplished using slings, immobilizers, casts, and traction, and surgical procedures to insert pins, wires, plates, and rods; for some hip fractures, the joint is replaced.

Neurological Disorders

Transient Ischemic Attacks

A transient ischemic attack (TIA) is a temporary interruption of blood flow to part of the brain, usually lasting no more than 24 hours. The cause is arteriosclerosis or spasm of the blood vessels. The symptoms can be inability to write or speak, sensations of pain or numbness, and loss of muscle control on one side of the body. Amnesia, inability to recognize familiar things, loss of balance, and a fall with or without a blackout are common.

The treatment depends on how many TIAs have occurred and which blood vessels are involved. Drugs that inhibit the formation of clots are prescribed. Surgical bypass of the obstructed vessels may be performed.

Cerebrovascular Accidents

A cerebrovascular accident (CVA) is also known as a "stroke." It may occur suddenly or over a period of time as a result of diminished blood supply to the brain (repeated TIAs). The person can suffer from impaired communication and sensory, perceptual, and motor function. Factors that predispose the elderly to strokes are arteriosclerosis and heart disease.

The signs and symptoms can be subtle; they include the following:

- Little memory lapses
- Sudden numbness in an extremity
- Difficulty in swallowing or speaking
- Some loss of vision in one eye
- Finding oneself on the floor, unable to get up, and not remembering the fall
- Sensory deficit, for example, burning oneself on a hot pan and not feeling it

Severe signs and symptoms follow occlusion of a large vessel; these are hemiplegia, quadriplegia, incontinence, sensory losses, and the major visual problem of being able to see only half of everything in the visual field.

The treatment depends on the symptoms and begins with assessing the damage. The patient can be in various stages of paralysis and helplessness. Long-term treatment can involve total care, speech therapy, and physical therapy. Visual retraining is often required. The rehabilitation period following a major stroke is long and intense. Family education and support are essential to the success of the program. The American Heart Association and the Sister Kenny Institute have a wealth of information on strokes, self-help, and rehabilitation.

Parkinson's Disease

Parkinson's disease is a progressive disease of the central nervous system in which there is faulty transmission of impulses from one neuron to another. Arteriosclerosis may be a factor in old age. A faint, constant tremor may be the first clue to the onset. The muscles gradually stiffen, and movement is slow and weak. With progression of the disease, the person walks with a shuffling gait and leans forward. Rigid muscles in the face and neck cause drooling, difficulty swallowing, and monotonous and slowed speech. The face becomes mask-like when the individual can not blink or smile. Increased tremors are evident in the classic "pill rolling" movement of the thumb hitting against the fingers.

Levodopa, or dopamine, is a drug currently used in treatment to help impulses get from one neuron to another and thereby relieve symptoms. People with Parkinson's disease must be protected from frustration and tension because these aggravate the symptoms. Nutritional therapy and physical therapy will help the person to lead a more normal life.

Diabetes Mellitus

Diabetes mellitus is a condition that results when the body cells are unable to use or store glucose due to lack of insulin. Normally, insulin is produced by the beta cells of the islets of Langerhans on the surface of the pancreas. Glucose is stored in the liver as glycogen and released when the body needs it for energy. Without adequate insulin to enable that glucose to pass through cell membranes, it accumulates in the bloodstream, a condition known as hyperglycemia. It spills over into the urine, and this is called glycosuria. Diabetes mellitus is treated by diet, oral hypoglycemics to reduce blood sugar, and insulin. Since a considerable amount of information is available on this disease, the nurse is referred to other sources for more details. The elderly diabetic presents a somewhat different picture than a diabetic who is younger.

The Older Diabetic

There are a number of factors that interfere with diagnosis and treatment of diabetes in the older person. Diagnosis is difficult because symptoms are often nonspecific: orthostatic hypotension, stroke, impotence, neuropathy, confusion, infection, and other symptoms are present. Older diabetics commonly have hyperglycemia without glycosuria. An older diabetic may have a normal fasting blood sugar and an elevated blood sugar for a couple of hours after a meal. Hypoglycemia, an abnormally low blood sugar, may be a greater threat because symptoms of this condition are atypical. The elderly diabetic may have decreased mental acuity, behavior disorders, poor sleep patterns with headaches, and slurred speech.

Anxiety and depression may hinder instruction about the disease. The elderly patient may feel that life is already too short and that diabetes will shorten it even more. Learning may be limited by impaired vision, hearing, speech, and mental status.

Oral hypoglycemics may interact with other drugs such as diuretics, antihypertensives, and thyroid preparations, all commonly taken by the older person. Eating habits are affected by poor dentition, tremors, arthritis, alterations in gastrointestinal function, and impaired mental function. In addition, an older person in bereavement might not want to cook or eat. Another problem is that older people exercise less and are less mobile than the average young person.

Dermatological Problems

Herpes Zoster

Herpes zoster, better known as "shingles," is an inflammation of a spinal ganglia. This condition is characterized by small clusters of vesicles or blisters along the pathway of the sensory nerves, most frequently around one side of the lower chest from posterior to anterior midline. Pain is usually burning, persistent and intense. After about one week the lesions crust. There is no known drug therapy for treatment other than analgesics and sedatives for relief of pain. Menthol camphor or calamine lotion applications are sometimes helpful.

Stasis Dermatitis

Venous stasis and edema in the lower extremities can cause poorly oxygenated tissue. The skin on the leg looks "dead" and scaly. Scratching and other trauma leads to ulcers. An Unnas boot made of zinc paste ointment is applied for one to two weeks over clean ulcers. Infected stasis ulcers are treated by controlling the infections with oral antibiotics and dressing the ulcer with bactericidal solutions.

Decubitus Ulcers

Decubitus ulcers are pressure sores that develop, usually over bony prominences, as a result of lack of oxygen to tissues. They are also known as bed sores. The skin eventually becomes necrotic and sloughs off. Aging people are susceptible to decubitus ulcers, or decubiti, because of fragile skin, poor nutrition, decreased sensations of pain and pressure, and conditions that cause edema and immobility (Fig. 8-1).

Decubitis ulcers develop in stages and can be treated accordingly.

Stage I — Skin is red but unbroken, and will not blanch or return to normal within 30 minutes. Swelling is present. Clean with pH-compatible soap and apply a therapeutic moisturizer and a transparent dressing to protect the area from friction. Op-Site is preferable.

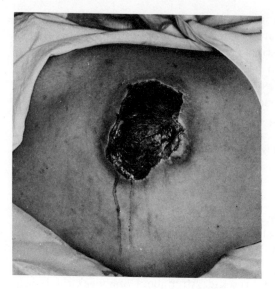

Figure 8–1. Elderly patients are susceptible to painful decubitus ulcers.

Stage II—There is loss of some skin, but not through dermis. The wound may appear as a blister. The wound base is moist, pink, and painful. There may be a white or yellow area of early dead tissue in wound bed.

Stage III—An open lesion, with penetration through the dermis, involves the subcutaneous tissue. The wound may be starting into fat and muscle. Necrotic tissue is possible and the wound base is not usually painful.

Stage IV—There is a deep penetrating wound, with involvement of fascia, muscle, and/or bone. The wound may include necrotic tissue, sinus tracts, drainage, and infection.

Cleansing and irrigating ulcers in stages II, III, and IV is done with normal saline or one-quarter-strength hydrogen peroxide. Where infection appears evident, agents such as Dakin's solution, Betadine, or acetic acid may be used. New tissue forms by granulation from the bottom up when the ulcer is kept clean and dead tissue is removed. Debridement or removal of the necrotic tissue is done in a number of ways:

- Transparent dressing is applied, usually Op-Site for minor debridement.
- For mechanical debridement, wet dressings are applied. When they are dry, they are removed and dead tissue comes off with them.
- Using a water pic, the force of water washes dead tissue away.

- For chemical debridement, special ointments are applied to dressings. Travase ointment is an example.
- Surgical debridement is another alternative.

Keeping further pressure off the ulcer is essential to the treatment. Using procedures to prevent decubitus ulcers is important (see Chap. 9).

Hematological Problems

Many older people are anemic, most commonly suffering from iron deficiency anemia. A poor diet is a major cause of anemia, and rheumatoid arthritis, diabetes, ulcers, infections, and cancer can be other causes. Pernicious anemia is caused by vitamin B_{12} deficiency. A folic acid deficiency results from a lack of fruits and vegetables in the diet. General signs of anemia are headaches, dizziness, fatigue, atrophy of the tongue, dry, stiff skin and thin, brittle hair, and fingernails. Prematurely white hair may be indicative of pernicious anemia. Anemias are treated by supplying the missing nutrient.

Eye Problems

Cataracts

A cataract is a clouding of the lens of the eye, which gradually loses its transparency. When blurring of vision becomes severe, vision in the affected eye is often described as "looking through milky water." Surgery to remove the lens and replace it with an implant is a highly successful treatment, usually done on an outpatient basis.

Glaucoma is another age-related condition (see Chap. 7).

Mental Disorders

Depression

Considering the losses and changes that occur with advancing age, it is not surprising that depression is extremely prevalent in older people. Although many persons are treated for depression throughout a lifetime, the condition can begin in old age. Since some of the symptoms are similar to those of dementia, the diagnosis of depression must be carefully made after a thorough assessment. Patients with depression lose interest

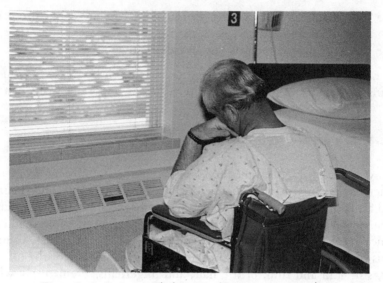

Figure 8-2. Patients with depression lose interest in everything.

in everything and every kind of activity (Fig. 8-2). They do not eat or sleep well. They suffer from fatigue, anorexia, weight loss, headaches, and constipation. A negative self-image is accompanied by guilt, remorse, and pessimism. At times a depressed person may be confused or exhibit poor judgment. Depression may lead to withdrawal, despair, and even suicide. Psychotherapy and antidepressant drugs are used in treatment.

Paranoia

Paranoia is marked by feelings of persecution. The paranoid individual is accusing and suspicious. In old age, paranoia is common — and with some valid reasons. When one can not see well or hear well, misconceptions of the behavior and motives of others is understandable. Poor health, limited finances, and the loneliness experienced by many older people promote paranoia. The stress of losing control over one's own affairs can also cause one to act as if others are taking advantage of him or her. When this happens, then there is someone to blame for what goes wrong.

Blaming others is also a way of preserving self-esteem. For example, it is easier to accuse someone of "changing things around" than it is to acknowledge that one can not remember where they put certain possessions. The negative attitude of society toward aging and the fraud and crimes of which older people are victims contribute to the malady. Treatment begins with trying to reduce the older person's feeling of insecurity.

Anxiety Reactions

Anxiety in older people causes a host of complaints and reactions. Fatigue, insomnia, restlessness, jittery behavior, an increase in pulse and blood pressure, changes in appetite, and a "nervous bladder" are only a handful of the signs of anxiety. Treatment depends on the cause.

Organic Brain Syndrome

Organic brain syndrome (OBS) is a general term applied to a set of symptoms due to abnormalities in structure and function of the brain. These abnormalities can be due to dysfunction or disease. The distinguishing feature of an OBS is cognitive loss: impairment of orientation, judgment, memory, comprehension, learning, and knowledge. Reversible brain syndromes are usually acute. Some of the causes are malnutrition, heart failure, brain tumors, and infection. Chronic syndromes are irreversible; these syndromes include the dementias.

Dementias

Dementia is a progressive decline in intellectual function. It is estimated that over three million people suffer with some type of dementia. The following are three causes of dementia in older adults:

Alzheimer's disease — This disease causes brain atrophy with plaques and tangles in the cortex. According to some sources, more than two million Americans and their families struggle with Alzheimer's disease.

Multi-infarct dementia — In this condition, there are many ischemic lesions and the occurrence of strokes.

Huntington's disease — This hereditary disease begins in middle age. Irregular and involuntary muscle movement occur.

Alzheimer's disease is the most common dementia. The Alzheimer's patient experiences behavior and personality changes in fairly predictable stages. One way of listing these is as follows:

STAGE I

Short-term memory loss
Gradual lack of interest in life
Can't remember nouns
Vague
Indifferent to social courtesies (will avoid people, groups)

STAGE II

Significant decline in memory
Difficulty with familiar tasks
Confuses day and night
Responds slowly
May complain of neglect
May deny problems
Loses things
Has trouble with directions
Self-neglect

STAGE III

Loses sense of time
Disoriented to place
Insomnia
Speech may ramble; incoherent
Motor ability deteriorates
Paranoid
Confused

STAGE IV

Incontinent of stool and urine
Mute
Extreme physical decline

Persons with Alzheimer's disease deteriorate at individual rates, but eventually they do become totally unable to care for themselves. They fight, throw things, run away, take off their clothes, and refuse care. The frustration and anguish for the family are difficult to bear. A definite diagnosis of Alzheimer's can only be made on autopsy. The brain will show atherosclerotic plaques and tangles of nerve fiber.

Treatment of a patient with Alzheimer's disease involves providing a safe environment with consistent routines, attention, contact with familiar things, and love. For example, sing with the patient if that will keep him quiet or under control. Drug therapy is in the experimental stage. Alzheimer's is a major health problem, and information on education and support groups is available from:

Alzheimer's Disease and Related
Disorders Association
70 E. Lake St
Chicago, IL 60601-5997

Cancer

Some facts about cancer in older people are as follows:

- Cancer is the second-leading cause of death.
- Cancer may go undetected because the symptoms are confused with other problems. For instance, rectal bleeding may be colon cancer, *not* hemorrhoids.
- Basal cell cancer, the *most common* skin cancer, occurs after age 40.
- Cancer is quite common throughout the gastrointestinal system, from the lip to the rectum.
- Cancer of the colon and rectum is the most common gastrointestinal cancer.
- Cancer of the lung is increasing.
- The occurrence of breast cancer in females increases with age.
- Cancer of the prostate is common in older men.
- Most people with cancer of the gallbladder are older.
- Myeloma, lymphosarcoma, and leukemia are prevalent forms of cancer.
- While elderly people generally have high pain thresholds, they *do* experience severe pain with cancer.

Treatment

As in younger people, treatment is based on the type of tumor, general condition of the patient, and patient preferences. Age should not be a major consideration.

Prevention

Routine health education for older people should include teaching the seven warning signs of cancer:

- Change in bladder and bowel habits
- Sore that will not heal
- Unusual bleeding or discharge
- Lump in breast or anywhere else
- Indigestion or difficulty in swallowing
- Marked change in wart or mole
- Hoarseness or a nagging cough

Advise the older person as follows:

- Do not smoke
- Avoid excessive intake of alcohol
- Eat a well-balanced diet; avoid eating food that is extremely hot, cold, or spicy
- Avoid prolonged exposure to the sun
- See the dentist if you have jagged teeth or poorly fitting dentures
- Difficulty in urinating should be checked by a physician
- Have a yearly physical examination, with colon and rectal exam and, if female, mammography

Summary

Physiological changes related to aging contribute to the development of disease and disorders in older people. The most important point to remember is that the symptoms of disease in older people can be very different and frequently less severe than in younger people. Cardiovascular disease is common, and one condition can often lead to another. For example, any disease that affects the efficiency of the heart can lead to congestive heart failure. Chronic obstructive pulmonary disease (COPD) is also common, and older people are at greater risk for pneumonia. Gastric distress is a sign of a number of disorders and requires substantial changes in diet. Older people are at a high risk for renal failure. Urinary tract infection is a major cause of fever in the elderly. Of the musculoskeletal conditions, arthritis is the most common. A cerebrovascular accident (CVA), or "stroke," is more common among older persons; the severity and treatment vary. The older diabetic may have nonspecific symptoms, making diagnosis difficult. Aging people are susceptible to decubitis ulcers, but they can often be prevented. Alzheimer's disease, which is marked by a progressive decline in intellectual function, has become a national health concern, with resources available for education and support.

Activities

1. Identify one symptom of each of the following diseases/problems and write a nursing measure or observation for a patient experiencing that problem:
   a. Emphysema
   b. Venous thrombosis
   c. Hiatal hernia
   d. Urinary tract infection

e. Arthritis

f. Congestive heart failure

g. Paranoia

2. Describe diabetes in words that an older person (a new diabetic) could understand.

3. How would you respond to the following questions if they were asked by an older person (remember communication skills, and suggest information the person might actually be seeking):

a. "What is a cataract?"

b. "How do they know if you have Alzheimer's?"

c. "What makes me anemic?"

d. "What are shingles?"

4. Choose one of the following and write a nursing care plan for a patient with that condition (include ADL and basic needs considerations):

a. COPD

b. Diverticulitis

c. Renal failure

d. Stress incontinence

e. CVA

f. Diabetes

g. Alzheimer's (advanced)

h. Pneumonia

Bibliography

Burnside I: Nursing and the Aged: A Self-Care Approach, 3rd ed. New York, McGraw-Hill, 1988

Ebersole P, Hess P: Toward Healthy Aging: Human Needs and Nursing Response, 2nd ed. St. Louis, CV Mosby, 1985

Eliopoulos C: Gerontological Nursing, 2nd ed. Philadelphia, JB Lippincott, 1987

Henderson M: Assessing the elderly, part 2: Altered presentations. Am J Nurs 85:1103–1106, 1985

Kaplan H, Sadock B (eds): Comprehensive Textbook of Psychiatry/IV, Vol I, 4th ed. Baltimore, Williams & Wilkins, 1985

Lipson L: Diabetes in the elderly: Diagnosis, pathogenesis, and therapy. Am J Med 80(suppl):10–21, 1986

Miller B: Osteoarthritis in the primary health care setting. Orthop Nurs 6:42–46, 1987

Patrick M et al: Medical–Surgical Nursing: Pathophysiological Concepts. Philadelphia, JB Lippincott, 1986

Rossman I: Clinical Geriatrics, 3rd ed. Philadelphia, JB Lippincott, 1987

Steinberg F (ed): Care of the Geriatric Patient in the Tradition of E. V. Cowdry, 6th ed. St. Louis, CV Mosby, 1983

9

Nursing Care of the Aging Person

Learning Objectives

When you complete this chapter, you should be able to:

1. Identify key factors in nursing assessment of the older patient from hospital admission to discharge.
2. Outline a nursing care plan for an immobile, hospitalized elderly patient that shows attention to all body systems.
3. Compare and contrast nursing care of the patient with dysphagia and the patient with aphasia.
4. List general points on positioning patients in bed.
5. Discuss the use of hearing aids as to the following:
   a. type
   b. insertion and removal
   c. problems
6. Explain the alternatives to giving food and fluids orally.
7. Describe the process of getting an elderly patient out of bed and into a geriatric chair.
8. Discuss safety measures used for patients who are at bed rest and for those whom the nurse assists in ambulating.
9. Identify causes of confusion in older hospitalized patients.
10. List facts about medications and their use in older people.
11. Identify special needs of older surgical patients.
12. Discuss psychological considerations in the care of hospitalized elderly people.
13. Describe the characteristics of nursing home care from the standpoints of the resident and the nurse.
14. Outline a nursing care plan for a dying older patient.

When an older person becomes sick or dependent, he or she can be a mystery to unravel, a human being with complex health problems and the potential for more due to age-related changes. There are a variety of diseases common in old age. Some are more likely to be treated in the hospital than others. Hospitalization itself can be a physically and psychologically traumatic experience for the older person. A long lifetime of experiences affects the older person's response to treatment and nursing care.

A young man may come to the hospital with a knee problem, a college degree, a new job, a girlfriend, and a fervent desire to play basketball and volleyball again as soon as possible. More than likely he will fear nothing beyond the "needles" he will get prior to surgery.

An old man may come to the hospital with a knee problem, high blood pressure, periodic insomnia resulting from three years as a prisoner of war, a wife, three married children, and four grandchildren. His fervent desire is that he will be able to get back to the gardening that was curtailed when his knee pain developed. He may be optimistic, mobile, cooperative, and generally in high spirits, but he may be secretly afraid that his other knee will also "give out" before too long. He may be concerned about the fact that he gets up to go to the bathroom a couple of times every night and that he may become constipated if he can not eat the food to which he is accustomed. What information will he volunteer and what will the nurse need to do to inspire his trust in order to obtain additional information? What kind of interactions will be therapeutic?

The nurse is continuously observing and evaluating the whole patient, although daily care is based on specific problems. Some of these are responses to hospitalization. This is where a nursing diagnosis is the guideline.

Discharge planning is also more complex. Needs of the patient and the family must be carefully assessed to determine what community resources may be needed. A nursing home may be a temporary or permanent solution to the need for continuing care. In the nursing home, routines and nursing responsibilities differ from those in the hospital because the goals are different.

Death is often the outcome of hospitalization for an older person. Hospice care, with its emphasis on living, can mean a peaceful, dignified death for that older person and lasting comfort for the family.

Nursing the older person who is acutely ill, dependent, debilitated or dying is a supreme challenge. The rewards are personal as well as professional, because the nurse has opportunities to acquire wisdom that will ease her own transition into the roles of aging.

The Older Patient in the Hospital

Hospital Admission

Admission to the hospital when one is sick is no longer an automatic process. More and more diagnostic tests are scheduled on an outpatient basis.

The diagnostic related groups system (DRGs) of reimbursement of medical expenses means that hospitals are only reimbursed a specific amount by Medicare. A certain number of days is allowed for a certain problem. Older patients scheduled for surgery may frequently enter the hospital the day of surgery and are discharged as soon as they can get in and out of bed without help (Fig. 9–1).

Advances in surgical techniques have increased the number of procedures done on an outpatient basis. "Short stay" units, in which postoperative patients remain only long enough to recover from anesthesia, are widespread.

Older people are frequently admitted to the hospital for these conditions:

- Congestive heart failure—evaluation and treatment plan
- Angina

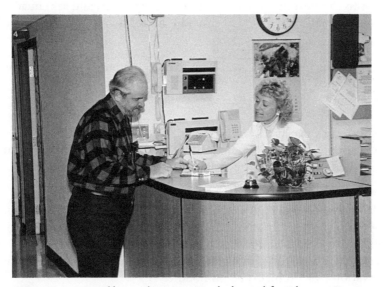

Figure 9–1. More older people are entering the hospital for "short stay" procedures (less than 24 hours).

- Pneumonia
- Gastrointestinal bleeding
- Pain, nausea, vomiting—symptoms of suspected bowel obstruction, cancer?
- Dehydration
- COPD
- CVA
- Septicemia
- Urinary tract infection
- Uncontrolled diabetes
- Nursing home placement
- Multiple symptoms that are incapacitating—could be cancer, onset of other disease, or drug related. One estimate is that 25% of hospital admissions in the 65+ age group are drug related.
- Fractures—usually hips
- Falls
- Scheduled surgery: total joint replacement, TUR, resection of tumor, neurological surgery, heart surgery

Initial Interview and Assessment

The fundamentals of interviewing and assessment were discussed in previous chapters. What the nurse needs to know in admitting the older person to the hospital is what to look for, listen for, and ask, in addition to routine questions, that will provide the following information:

- Reason for admission
- Medical history that will help identify potential problem areas and chronic conditions that will need attention
- Health education needs
- Fears and anxieties
- Patient's expectations and goals
- Patient's support system and who the primary contacts will be when information needs to be validated or completed
- Where to begin discharge planning

With this knowledge, the nurse is able to plan *realistic* nursing care. For example, if the patient is slightly overweight and tells the nurse that she hates to exercise and is "too old anyway," it is realistic to plan to supervise and assess *all* postoperative ambulation and to make continuous observations for problems of immobility.

Before the nurse begins the interview, she should realize that anxiety may interfere with what the patient tells her and what the patient hears.

During the interview, the nurse must allow time for repetition and validation. Here is where her knowledge of normal aging immediately becomes valuable. An older person needs more time to respond to questions because reaction time is slower. Another factor is that the patient may have numerous problems and a lot of years to remember. By careful listening and by drawing the patient out, the nurse can begin to assess the level of understanding early in the interview. When the patient has a known or suspected dementia, this will not be possible.

Whatever the older patient tends to dwell on, a symptom or other subject, is significant for some reason and the nurse must learn what that reason is. If it has to do with any of the patient's health problems, a good question to ask is, "What has the doctor told you?" Patients offer some common responses and cues, and an interview may take one of a number of directions (see the display, "Admission Interview Highlights").

If a fall has occurred, the patient may complain of dizziness or headaches during the interview. Age-related changes, diseases, and poor safety precautions are responsible for the high incidence of falls in older people. Older people can and do fall anywhere: at home, on the street, in stores, and in health care institutions.

Depending on the situation and the patient's condition after a fall, some of the following questions can be asked:

- "Why do you think you fell?"
- "Did you fall forward, backward, sideways or did you slide to a sitting position?"
- "Do you remember falling? Or did you wake up and find yourself on the floor?"
- "Did you hit your head? Black out?"
- "How long were you on the floor?"
- "Before you fell were you dizzy, short of breath, feeling pain, weak, or lightheaded? Was your heart pounding?"
- "Was any part of your body numb?"
- "Did you lose control of your bladder or bowels after you fell?"
- "Were you sick to your stomach?"
- "Were you able to get up alone? If not, how did you call for help?"
- "Has this ever happened to you before?"
- "Did you slip? Was the floor wet or your shoes slippery?"
- "Do you have new glasses? Were you wearing glasses?"
- "Was the lighting good? Could you see where you were going?"
- "Were you using, or had you been using, a cane or walker?"
- "Was there anything in your pathway?"
- "Had you just taken any medication?"
- "Where do you hurt?"

Admission Interview Highlights

Patient: A.H. is a 71-year-old female who is being admitted with dizziness, some numbness in her arms and pain in her wrists.

Patient	Nurse
1. Immediately asks if her B.P. is too high. 162/88. "My father had a stroke when he was only 54."	*Ask:* What is your B.P. usually? *Consider:* Patient concerned about having a CVA? May need to obtain family history first and assess need for instruction about strokes and need for emotional support.
2. Repeats symptoms of pain in wrists and numbness in arms a couple times. Rubbing them.	Inspect arms. Check R.O.M. *Ask:* How long have you had this? What makes it feel better or worse? What does it prevent you from doing? What were you doing when it started? *Consider:* If discussion of father's stroke comes up again, a fear has been identified.
3. Vague about dizziness. Happens at "different times." Is not dizzy now.	*Consider:* Dizziness may be normal? Is patient denying it? *Ask:* Did you fall recently? If yes, how? Did you trip or wake up on the floor? Do you have new glasses? Need new glasses? Have a hearing problem? Headaches? Patient will need to be observed at various times for evidence of dizziness. Ask her to report it.
4. "Look at these wrists. My neighbor says I have arthritis."	*Consider:* 3rd time wrists were mentioned. Does patient fear arthritis and the dependency it may bring?

(continued)

Admission Interview Highlights (*Continued*)

Patient	Nurse
	Ask: Did your wrists and arms start bothering you at the same time? Symptoms may be unrelated. Ask about other joints and inquire into activities and anything she's had to give up doing.
5. Past medical history includes "blood clots in legs."	*Consider:* Need to investigate this thoroughly to determine if *prevention* of thrombophlebitis and observation for pulmonary embolism will be a priority if patient spends much time in bed.
6. Has been a widow for six years and lives in a duplex. Son and daughter-in-law live on other side: Both work at jobs. Patient came to hospital from doctor's office, via a neighbor.	*Consider:* Information on dizziness is vague. More information may be provided by son. Need to know this as TIAs may need to be ruled out.

While asking the above questions, assess the following:

- Check vital signs.
- Inspect skin for lacerations, redness, and bruises.
- Note mental status and any evidence of slurred speech when getting answers to questions.
- Palpate head and spinal column for painful areas, moving the patient as little as possible.
- Ask the patient to move arms and legs and compare one extremity to the other.
- Check hand grasps; note any weakness or inequality.
- Note any tremors.
- Check the pupils for reaction to light: are they equal? Describe.

Remember these points:

- Bruises may not develop for 24 hours.
- Pain and stiffness may increase.
- Changes in mental status, ability to move, vision, vital signs, plus restlessness, headache, nausea, and vomiting may be signs of intercranial pressure caused by bleeding or swelling.

Functional assessments should be done when the patient is admitted, in order to help in setting realistic goals and planning for discharge. Was the patient living independently? Was some assistance in the home necessary? Was the patient in a dependent situation; for example, did the patient come from a nursing home?

Daily Observations

Every day the nurse makes observations and plans care based on the following:

- The reason the patient is in the hospital. For example, a patient with congestive heart failure must be observed for increased edema in legs.
- Age-related problems that the patient describes or the nurse can diagnose. For example, if dry skin is observed, the patient on bed rest must have backrubs and position changes every three hours.
- Prevention of problems that might occur because of the patient's individual ability. For example, a fragile, 82-year-old, 100-pound woman is getting out of bed for the first time in three days. To prevent undue fatigue and weakness, she should be allowed to rest before she makes the attempt.
- Prevention of problems that might occur because of the patient's personality. For example, a 76-year-old man who will not accept help with his meals and will eat only one pea at a time should get his meal trays first, if necessary, so he gets adequate nourishment.
- The reality of early discharge. For example, an 80-year-old woman, who has had a surgical pinning of a fractured hip, has been living alone. She may need physical therapy or supervised ambulation in her home or two to three weeks in a nursing home for therapy.

Practical Use of the Nursing Diagnosis

In caring for aging patients, the nurse will be guided by multiple nursing diagnoses in planning the details of individual patient care.

Working with the Nursing Diagnosis

| 79-Year-Old Man
4 Days Postoperative
Knee Surgery | 79-Year-Old Woman
with Bone Cancer |

Nursing Diagnosis

Sleep pattern disturbance related to nocturia (age-related change)

Sleep pattern disturbance related to pain, anxiety, depression, drugs

Plan

1. Decaffeinated coffee for supper.
2. Restrict fluids after 6 p.m. Inform patient this may reduce number of trips to bathroom.
3. Leave bathroom light on.
4. Put walker next to his bed.
5. Be certain call light is within reach. Request that he use it when he gets up so you can check how safely he ambulates.

1. Give pain medication as appropriate.
2. When settling patient for sleep, spend extra time with her.
3. Offer warm milk if tolerated.
4. Check patient every one to two hours. If she's awake, touch her hand or arm. Stand by her bed a few minutes.
5. Offer position changes and backrub.
6. Say: "I will stay with you a while," or ask: "What can I do to make the night easier?"

A nursing diagnosis states a patient problem and the possible reasons for its existence (see Chap. 2). This is how nursing care is planned for the *individual* patient (see the display, "Working with the Nursing Diagnosis").

Nursing Care

The changes related to aging occur throughout the entire body and are often similar to signs and symptoms of disease, so the nurse must observe and care for the older patient as a *complete* person rather than as a patient with a disease or problem. Thus, hands-on care should be based on nursing actions and observations for a 24-hour period.

Care and Observations: Bath and Personal Hygiene

Whether the nurse is assisting an older patient with personal care or giving a complete bath, a head-to-toe inspection must be made. The nurse must ask questions and make observations about comfort, progress, and potential problems while performing nursing actions.

How Did the Patient Sleep?

Determining whether the patient slept well should be the first consideration of the morning. How the patient slept can affect appetite, physical stamina, disposition, and response to care and treatment all day. The patient who is not well rested lacks the ability to concentrate. Although a 7 a.m. report may *say* that the patient had a good night, this must be verified with that patient. The patient may have slept fitfully, had disturbing dreams, or experienced distress that was not reported for either of two reasons. One, the patient may be a "poor" sleeper normally, and two, he or she may have been reluctant to "bother" the nurse. When the patient does not finish breakfast, is disinterested in being fed, or cannot seem to start a bath, the nurse should be suspicious of a sleepless night. A short rest period before the bath and a mid-morning snack may be indicated.

Suggest that the patient stretch arms and legs, slowly at first, and move feet and hands to increase circulation. The patient should also do head rotations and shrug the shoulders. If the patient cannot help himself, the nurse should move the feet back and forth, gently, to stretch the leg muscles, and then flex the wrists and elbows. This is the instruction: "We can help your circulation by doing this, and later it will be easier for you to move around."

The personality factor of being a "morning person" or an "afternoon person" is a psychological consideration in care of the total person. It can have a profound effect on the nurse–patient relationship at this time. Some individuals do not function as well in the morning as they do in the afternoon. They prefer to sleep late when possible and skip breakfast, and they may "come alive" late in the day. When they enter the hospital this does not change. Although many older persons are early risers, they may still prefer to take their morning activities slowly. The nurse should be aware of this fact, having gleaned this information from the admission interview. "Do you usually bathe in the morning?" and "Do you eat breakfast?" are questions that can be asked any time. A family member or spouse can validate the answers.

Morning Care

The need for a complete bath or shower daily should be determined by the condition of the patient's skin, the presence of body odors, and the patient's preference, if possible. The patient who does not wish to be bathed, but who needs a bath must be approached with tact:

> "Mr. J, I can only tell if your skin is staying healthy if I can see it while we get you bathed and rubbed."
> "Bathing is good for your circulation."
> "Kidneys don't work as well when you are in bed a lot and bladder infections are easier to get. Bathing can help prevent them."

Sometimes patients make jokes such as, "Who cares how I look?" The nurse responds: "I care because I care about you, and I know you will feel better."

Skin Condition

Observe the condition of the patient's skin, expecting some dryness. Look behind the ears, under the breasts, and under any folds of fat, and inspect the gluteal fold and the perineum. Check the skin over bony prominences and between the toes. Report and document redness, bruises, breaks in skin, sores, or lumps; skin tags or lesions that appear irritated must also be noted. A lotion rub to the back, buttocks, elbows, and knees should be routine following the bath. A rash, especially on pressure areas, may indicate that the hospital linen or soap is irritating the patient's skin. Standard hospital procedures for dealing with this problem include special soaps and linens. A rash may also indicate a reaction to medication, so all rashes must be reported. Skin turgor is tested by gently pinching the skin. Poor turgor, or lack of firmness, may be a sign that the patient is dehydrated. Make a note of this, so that oral fluids can be encouraged or intravenous therapy begun. Special lotions, powders, or creams that belong to the patient should be used whenever possible.

Cyanosis of the nailbeds is a sign of poor circulation and should be noted. When fingernails or toenails need trimming, they should be trimmed or filed straight across the nail. Diabetics and patients with circulatory problems should not have their nails trimmed without a physician's order, and then, perhaps, only by a podiatrist.

Special Mattresses and Pads

Specially equipped beds for immobile patients and mattresses and pads that relieve pressure are numerous and vary with institutions. They are valuable for immobile patients. A turning sheet is an extra drawsheet under the patient that has been folded in half to make a square. With a turning sheet, or "lifter," a patient can be lifted to one side of the bed and turned on the opposite side, as well as moved to the head or foot of the bed (Fig. 9–2). The nurse should always avoid dragging a patient across sheets or pulling him to a sitting position.

The Head and Neck

Encourage older people to comb their own hair because it provides arm exercise. Ask how the scalp feels and inspect it for redness, scaling, or lesions. Ask the patient about the possibility of applying mineral oil to an itchy scalp.

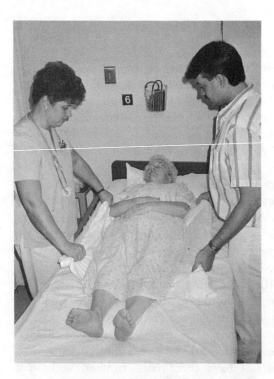

Figure 9–2. A turning sheet, or "lifter," makes it easier to move the patient with limited mobility.

Mouth and Throat

Routine oral hygiene is appropriate for patients with normal swallowing (see Chap. 6). Report and document any sores or white patches on mucous membranes or tongue. A major mouth and throat problem is loss of control of the muscles of the tongue, mouth, or pharynx due to a stroke. The patient may have dysphagia, which is difficulty chewing and difficulty swallowing. Decreased ability to cough, expectorate, and clear the airway are other symptoms of impaired muscle function. Nursing care for this kind of patient includes preventing aspiration of food and fluids into lungs:

- If the gag reflex is absent, the patient should not wear dentures because of the possibility of choking on them. Testing the gag reflex can be done by gently touching the back of the patient's throat with a tongue blade.
- Suction equipment for the oral and nasal passages should be left in the room at all times.
- When the patient is eating, being fed, drinking, and taking medications, the head of the bed should be elevated as high as the patient can tolerate.
- Coughing and deep breathing should be encouraged, when possible, every four hours. Depending on the patient's condition, the nurse may need to use oral suction following the patient's coughing attempts.
- When the gag reflex is present and the patient responds to verbal stimuli, the nurse may apply water with a swab or drip water into the mouth from a straw to provide fluids (Fig. 9–3).
- If gag is present, but the patient has a problem with water, try semisolids such as pudding.
- Note the condition of the tongue and mucous membrane.

The Aphasic Patient

Aphasia is the inability to use or understand language. This is a neurological disorder which, in older patients, is usually the result of a stroke. Aphasia is most often a mixture of communication deficits. These deficits include:

- Slow speech
- Incorrect speech
- Incorrect words and sounds

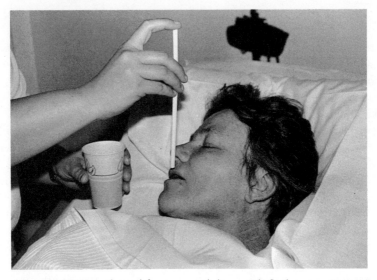

Figure 9–3. Water dropped from a straw helps provide fluids to a patient with dysphagia.

- Inability to understand speech or writing
- Persistent repetition of a word or phrase, called perseveration
- Trouble naming objects

The patient may or may not be aware of the difficulties he is having. The patient who is aware is frustrated and depressed. Emotional lability is very common in stroke patients.

When caring for the patient with aphasia, the nurse can communicate with the patient according to the extent of his disability:

- *Talk* to the patient while you work; explain what you are doing. Do this for all conscious patients.
- Use a normal tone of voice and speak slowly.
- Use short sentences.
- Ask simple questions with yes or no answers.
- Ignore profanity; it is part of the response to the deficit.
- Make no attempts to correct the patient's mistakes.
- Share the patient's frustration and do not pretend to understand when you do not understand. Say, "How frustrated you must get when you want to talk to me."
- Point, gesture, write. Work out a system for the patient to use in responding, for example, "Squeeze my hand once for yes."
- Remember that no may mean yes.

- Praise success.
- Communication comes more easily if the patient is not tired.
- Don't rush the patient through a response.

Vision

Does the patient wear glasses? Glasses should be kept clean, and the patient should be wearing them as necessary. Place meal trays, water pitchers, bathing utensils, boxes of tissue, and other items where the patient can see them. Ask the patient about the amount of lighting needed to see. Is there a glare with window blinds open or from ceiling lights? Adjust the environment accordingly. Ask the patient if filling out menus is difficult and, if so, offer assistance.

Hearing

If the patient has a hearing deficit, there should be a sign at the head of the bed as well as directions on file about what works to communicate with this patient. Is one ear more affected than the other? Does the patient have a hearing aid? The nurse should know how hearing aids work, how to put them on and remove them, and how to clean them.

Hearing Aids

There are different types of hearing aids (see Fig. 9–4):

A. The in-the-canal aid is contained entirely in an earmold worn in the ear canal.
B. The in-the-ear aid is contained entirely in an earmold worn in the cradle of the ear.
C. The behind-the-ear aid is worn behind the ear with a plastic tube leading to an earmold worn in the canal.
D. The body-worn aid is clipped to the wearer's clothing, with a cord leading to a button-like earmold worn in the cradle of the ear.
E. The eyeglass aid is built into the wearer's eyeglasses, with a plastic tube leading to an earmold worn in the ear canal.

IMPORTANT—No matter what type of hearing aid your patient wears, it is crucial to remember the following points:

1. *Before you start to place any aid,* make sure you determine if the hearing aid is for the LEFT ear or the RIGHT ear.
2. Make sure the aid is turned OFF, if there is an ON–OFF switch.

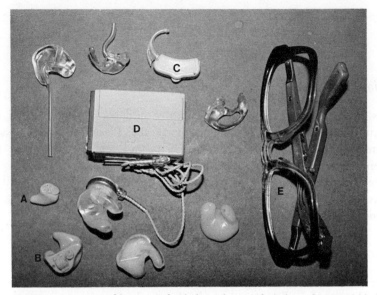

Figure 9–4. Types of hearing aids: (A) in-the-canal, *(B)* in-the-ear, *(C)* behind the ear, *(D)* body-worn, *(E)* eyeglass aid. Also shown are ear-mold models.

On some models, the ON–OFF function is regulated by opening or closing the battery door. In that case, the battery door should be closed, but *the volume control should be turned all the way down.*

3. *Before removing any aid,* the volume should be turned all the way *down* and the aid turned OFF wherever possible.

In-the-Canal Aid

To place the aid in the ear, follow these steps:

1. Insert the tapered end of the aid first. (The volume control should always face out.) Then carefully work the aid into the patient's ear canal, using a gentle twisting motion. It should fit snugly, yet comfortably. Do *not* force the aid too deeply into the ear canal.
2. On some models, the ON–OFF switch is built into the volume control. Twist the control forward, toward the front of the patient's head, and the aid will click ON. Once the aid is ON—and with the volume setting still all the way *down*—start talking to your patient in a normal tone of voice. Gradually turn the volume *up* until he can hear and understand comfortably.

To remove the aid from the ear, follow these steps:

1. Unseat the aid from the ear canal by placing your thumb just below the ear and pushing up and in. Once the aid is loose, remove it by using your thumb and index finger.
2. Do *not* remove the aid by pulling the volume control switch or the battery door.

In-the-Ear Aid

To place the aid in the ear, follow these steps:

1. Insert the extended canal portion of the aid first. (The volume control should always face out.) Then carefully work the aid into the cradle of the patient's ear, using a gentle twisting motion. Be sure it feels secure in the ear.
2. If there is an ON – OFF switch, turn it ON. With the volume still all the way *down*, start talking to your patient in a normal tone of voice. Gradually turn the volume *up* until he can hear and understand comfortably. Remember, always increase the volume by turning the control toward the front of the patient's head.

To remove the aid from the ear, follow these steps:

1. Gently loosen the aid from the top, lifting it up and out of the ear at the same time. Use the handy fingernail notches provided.
2. Do *not* remove the aid by pulling the volume control knob or the battery holder.

Behind-the-Ear Aid

To place the aid in the ear, follow these steps:

1. Place the aid over your patient's ear, making sure the earmold hangs free with no twists or kinks in the tubing.
2. Carefully insert the tapered end of the earmold into your patient's ear. Then gently twist the earmold into the cradle of the ear until it fits snugly. (For canal-type earmolds, place the long canal portion securely into the ear canal.) It will help if you pull down on the earlobe with your free hand and, at the same time, push up and in gently on the bottom of the earmold. It is important to get a good, tight fit; otherwise, "feedback" (whistling) may occur.
3. Turn the aid ON. With the volume still all the way *down*, start talking to your patient in a normal tone of voice. Gradually turn the volume *up* until he can understand comfortably.

To remove the aid from the ear, follow these steps:

1. Gently loosen the upper portion of the earmold, lifting it up and out at the same time. (Remove canal-type earmolds by gripping the bottom portion of the earmold in the cradle and pulling gently.)
2. Do *not* remove the earmold by pulling the plastic sound tube.

Eyeglass Aid

The hearing aid may be enclosed in the left or right temple of the eyeglasses or in both temples to help hearing in both ears. Each aid will be attached to an earmold designed to fit into the patient's ear cradle (and, in some cases, ear canal).

To place the aid in the ear, follow these steps:

1. Slip the eyeglass hearing aid on your patient as you would any ordinary pair of glasses.
2. Make sure the earmold(s) hang(s) free with no twists or kinks in the tubing.
3. Carefully insert the tapered end of the earmold into your patient's ear. Then gently twist the upper portion of the earmold into the cradle of the ear until it fits snugly. (For canal-type earmolds, place the long canal portion securely into the ear canal.) It will help if you pull down on the earlobe with your free hand and, at the same time, push up and in gently on the bottom of the earmold. It is important to get a good, tight fit; otherwise, feedback may occur.
4. Turn the aid ON, if necessary to do so. With the volume still all the way *down*, start talking to your patient in a normal tone of voice. Gradually turn the volume *up* until he or she can understand comfortably. If the patient has an aid for each ear, start with the less affected ear first; then repeat the process for the other ear.

To remove the aid from the ear, follow these steps:

1. Gently loosen the upper portion of the earmold, lifting it up and out at the same time. (Remove canal-type earmolds by gripping the bottom portion of the earmold in the cradle and pulling it gently.)
2. Do *not* remove the earmold by pulling the plastic sound tube.
3. Use both hands to remove the eyeglass hearing aid just as you would an ordinary pair of glasses.

Body-Worn Aid

To place the aid in the ear, follow these steps:

1. Clip the aid to the patient's clothing. (Try to keep it as far away from the ear as possible.)
2. Guide the cord and receiver button/earmold assembly to the ear.
3. Hold the button/earmold between your thumb and forefinger and insert the tapered end carefully into the ear canal. Then gently twist the upper portion of the earmold into the cradle of the patient's ear until it fits snugly. It will help if you pull down on the patient's earlobe with your free hand and, at the same time, push up and in gently on the bottom of the earmold. It is important to get a good, tight fit; otherwise, feedback may occur.
4. Turn the aid ON. With the volume still all the way *down*, start talking to your patient in a normal tone of voice. Gradually turn the volume *up* until he can understand comfortably.

To remove the aid from the ear, follow these steps:

1. Take hold of the button/earmold with your thumb and forefinger and gently loosen it, twisting it slightly toward the rear and lifting up and out at the same time.
2. Do *not* remove the earmold by pulling the cord.
3. Carefully disengage the aid from your patient's clothing.

Proper Care of a Hearing Aid

- A hearing aid should never be left on a windowsill, or on a table exposed to direct sunlight, or on hot surfaces such as radiators or heaters.
- Never use hair spray or medicinal spray while the patient is wearing a hearing aid.
- Never expose a hearing aid to steam or vapor of any kind.
- Never get a hearing aid wet; and never attempt to clean it with liquid.
- Never handle a hearing aid carelessly or drop it. Although hearing aids will take a considerable amount of everyday wear, they are still very delicate instruments that should be protected from unnecessary blows.
- Keep the earmold clean. Make sure wax is not accumulating in the canal tip. If clogged, the earmold should be cleaned *very carefully* with a special tool available from your local hearing aid dispenser.

Do not use pencils, scissors, tweezers, or toothpicks to remove wax. It is possible to wash gently the earmolds for behind-the-ear, eyeglass, and body-worn aids only in a mild soap-and-water solution —but *only* if the tubing is first gently disconnected from the body of the aid.

When the Hearing Aid Does Not Work

PROBLEM-SOLVING CHECKLIST

1. Be sure the aid is turned ON.
2. Be sure the battery is inserted and functioning properly. If a hearing aid "goes dead" quickly, the battery is probably no longer functioning. (A battery can stop functioning very quickly.) Before replacing a battery, it is important to make sure that the new battery is exactly the same type as the old one. Sometimes batteries appear similar, but they are different. If any doubt exists, check the number on the old battery. Hearing aids have a flip-open door or removable battery compartment. To replace a battery, open the compartment so that the battery is fully exposed. Notice which way the battery is resting in the compartment. Turn the aid over so that the old battery falls out into the palm of your hand. Place the new battery in the compartment. As a rule, the positive side of the battery should face up. The smaller end of the battery, the negative side, will generally face down in the compartment. Some new batteries can be defective. If you put in a fresh battery and the aid still does not function correctly, try another battery before attempting anything else.
3. Be sure the volume control is not turned too low for proper hearing.
4. Be sure the plastic sound tubing is not cracked, broken, or twisted. Be sure it does not have a loose connection and that it has no water in it. For body-aids, be sure the cord is functioning properly and that it is not shorting out.
5. Feedback may be caused by an improper fit of the ear mold. If the earmold seems to be inserted correctly and the feedback continues, a hearing aid specialist should be called.

All information about hearing aids courtesy of Beltone Electronic Corporation, Chicago, Illinois.

Pain: Nursing Implications

Although older people have decreased sensations of pain, they still experience pain. Their attitudes about pain affect their response. An older patient may be stoic, having come to expect pain as part of living. Many persons develop a higher pain tolerance over the years. Sometimes these are patients who do not want to "bother" anyone. Restlessness, clenched fists, grimacing, rigidity, anxiety, depression, and lack of appetite may be nonverbal signs of pain. Some patients become unusually quiet and appear apprehensive when they are having severe pain.

If possible, the patient should be asked to *describe* and *pinpoint* the pain. Ask questions: Is it a new pain? An old pain? If it's an old pain, is it better or worse? How long has it been there? Did some movement or other occurrence cause this pain? The pain belongs to the patient, who is the only one who knows exactly how it feels.

Prescribed medications for pain must be administered judiciously. Older people cannot tolerate narcotics well. Non-narcotic analgesics in combination with small doses of narcotics may be very effective and may reduce the risk of side-effects of confusion, weakness, dizziness, depressed respirations, nausea, and vomiting.

Nursing measures to control pain include backrubs, positional changes, gentle exercises to increase circulation, and deep breathing. A cool, wet cloth on the head eases a headache and makes other pain more tolerable. Darkening the room and playing soft, restful music when possible creates a soothing environment.

Listening to the patient and touching or holding the patient's hand help reduce anxiety and pain. Remember that pain is intensified by fear; often the fear is of not knowing what is happening or what is going to happen. The nurse must be sensitive to this in interactions with older patients at all times.

Positioning

Patients who are partially immobile, such as a new surgical patient or one with an affected extremity, must be repositioned at least every three hours. Patients who are totally immobile need position changes every two hours. Assessment of the skin at these times will determine if more frequent positioning is needed. For a patient who can help himself, an overhead bed frame with a trapeze is a useful device.

From head to toe, correct and frequent positioning will induce relaxation and prevent muscle strain and skin breakdown. For immobile patients, proper positioning will prevent contractures, nerve damage, and circulatory impairment.

Head Pillows

A small pillow under the head and neck of a patient on long-term bedrest will help prevent a flexion contracture of the neck. Large pillows under the head must be placed down under the shoulders for adequate neck and shoulder support.

Immobile patients should have small pillows or folded towels placed in the axillae and changed daily with the bath. Prolonged contact of skin against skin causes skin breakdown from perspiration.

Side-Lying or Lateral Position

A strict side-lying position is difficult to maintain because old shoulders become painful from the pressure, and circulation of the arm will be impaired. The hand will feel cool to the touch and the patient will complain, if able, of numbness, tingling, or pain. It is preferable to pull the lower shoulder and arm all the way out and place a pillow lengthwise to support both lower arms in a slightly flexed position. The top shoulder should always be supported by a pillow. There should be a pillow placed between the knees. The peroneal nerve lies about two inches below the head of the fibula and close to the bone on the lateral side of the leg. This nerve is susceptible to compression, with symptoms of pain, numbness, or tingling down the side of the leg or on the top of the foot. The patient who can not express such symptoms is at risk for nerve damage; this is a key reason why immobile patients must be turned so often.

Arm Position

When the patient is positioned on the back, pillows can be placed under the arms with the arms in positions that "appear" comfortable, across the chest, lower on the abdomen, or out to the sides. *The tips of the elbows should be visible.* If they are not, there is pressure on the ulnar nerve. The ulnar nerve passes through the elbow joint on the ulnar, or little-finger, side of the arm. When this nerve is compressed, the patient who is alert will complain of numbness and tingling of the ring finger and little finger and of pain in the hand and lower arm. Paralysis of this nerve is a complication that can occur in a matter of hours if pressure is not relieved.

Leg Position

The knee gatch should *not* be elevated. Pillows should not be used under legs because they "bunch" under the knees when patients move their legs and the popliteal space, with the nerves and blood vessels, is compressed. Venous return is slowed and the patient is at risk for thrombophlebitis. If pillows are used, they should be placed lengthwise. The heels should be off the bed. When the patient's legs are straight, a folded bath blanket placed under the legs from the Achilles tendon to above the popliteal space will keep the heels off the bed. Heels need special observation when repositioning patients because heels are subject to pressure every time a patient tries to help himself. Even with vigilant attention, they tend to come to rest on the bed more than they should. A heel that is likely to break down will look like pink parchment.

If the head of the patient's bed must be elevated for extended periods of time, bear in mind the risk of thrombophlebitis and inspect the legs with each change of position.

General Rules

- Flexors are usually stronger than extensors, and positions of slight flexion will be more comfortable. However, flexion contractures are a hazard of immobility which underlines the importance of position changes. Range-of-motion exercises, moving the joints within the limits of mobility and comfort, should be performed with positioning.
- When trying to determine if a patient is comfortable, put yourself in his position. One does not need to lie down to do this: turning the head, twisting the back, or holding an extremity in a position similar to that of the patient can be extremely enlightening.
- Never allow a patient to remain in the same position for more than three hours.
- In positioning an extremity, support adjacent joints. For example, if you elevate the lower arm on a pillow, support the elbow.
- Take into consideration the lifelong sleep habits of the patient. If he is able to tell you how he is most comfortable, position him accordingly whenever possible. For example, a patient who says he could never sleep on his back may be positioned on the right side for three hours, on the back for one hour, and then on the left side for three hours.
- Edematous limbs need elevation. Observe the amount of swelling and check for pitting. To do this, gently make an indentation with the thumb in the edema near a bony prominence and note if, and how long, the indentation remains.
- Immobile limbs, "hanging" down, become edematous, therefore they must be elevated as necessary and observed carefully.

- Extremities in casts and dressings also require elevation, higher than the heart. An exception to this is a hanging arm cast for a fractured humerus. The color, temperature, motion, and sensation of the fingers or toes on the affected limb must be assessed and documented according to hospital routine. This assessment must be done on *each* digit and includes the following observations:
  Observing color
  Feeling skin (temperature)
  Asking patient to flex, extend, and move it in all directions
  Gently pinching and asking if and what the patient can feel
- A trochanter roll can be helpful in relieving pressure on the buttocks (Fig. 9–5). Fold a drawsheet or bath blanket into a three-foot square. Turn the patient on one side. Place the folded linen under the patient and under one of the patient's buttocks. As the patient is turned back, roll the square *under* and toward the buttocks, as far as necessary to elevate slightly one side, relieving the pressure of one buttock.
- Doughnuts and rubber rings merely shift pressure from one point to another and should be avoided. Transparent dressings, such as Op-Site, applied to high-risk areas such as elbows and heels is preferable.

Bowel Functioning: Preventing Problems

Older persons who come to the hospital with well-established routines for preventing or coping with constipation need to have those routines

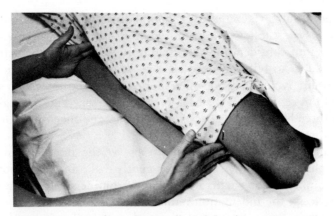

Figure 9–5. Use of a trochanter roll can help relieve pressure on the buttocks.

worked into their hospital days whenever feasible. Shortened hospital stays make it difficult for the nurse to instruct and guide an older patient in the formation of new habits. Tests and surgical procedures alter eating habits, cause pain and discomfort, and disrupt elimination patterns in general.

Careful attention to providing privacy and comfort when the patient is on a bedpan, commode, or toilet can prevent problems. Warming a bedpan with hot water, drying it, and applying powder to the sitting surface make it easier to sit on. Commodes must be a comfortable height. Patients who are weak and in pain need to be positioned on toilets and commodes so they are not clutching bars and supports because this makes it hard to relax and concentrate on the task at hand.

When the patient's condition permits, encourage liberal amounts of what the patient likes to drink, and help the patient select menu items high in fiber.

The nurse must be aware of all the possible causes of constipation (see Chap. 8) in the older patient and plan nursing actions that will prevent or modify problems for individual patients.

A patient with prolonged constipation, or one who goes from constipation to diarrhea, must be checked for a fecal impaction. Even if occasional diarrhea is normal for a particular patient, when that patient is in the hospital it must be investigated. Diarrhea may be caused by dietary factors or as a side-effect of medication. Anxiety can also be a cause. These possibilities must be ruled out. Diarrhea can be a symptom of another disorder, so it should be reported to the physician.

The Urinary Tract: Preventing and Detecting Problems

The color and odor of the urine should be noted daily because urinary tract infections often develop in older people who are hospitalized. Cloudy, foul-smelling urine is a danger signal. Older patients must get adequate fluids, but if their condition necessitates fluid restriction, this will be so stated in physician's orders. Those patients who are not capable of, or willing to, protest are commonly offered juices that the well-meaning nurse likes to drink or that are available in the unit refrigerator. If the patient can not choose, a family member should be consulted as to the patient's preferences.

The voiding habits of the older patient must be noted on admission for baseline information. This will make evaluation of urinary function more accurate. For instance, if the patient is having surgery, the nurse needs to know if it is normal for that patient to void often and in approximately what amounts. Otherwise it may be hard to decide whether or not the patient has urinary retention with overflow if he is voiding frequently in small amounts in the early postoperative period. When a patient has an indwelling catheter, hospital procedures for care must be strictly observed.

The Incontinent Patient

The older patient who is aware of his incontinence suffers distress and embarrassment. Even with any decrease in the sense of smell, that person knows he has an offensive odor and he is acutely conscious of the reactions of others. When incontinence is temporary due to the effect of medications, treatment, or environmental circumstances, the patient will require emotional support to "weather" this affliction. Cleanliness is of utmost importance. The perineal area and buttocks must be observed for rash or redness. Applying cornstarch to this type of rash is suggested. Disposable pads can be placed over the drawsheet with the instruction, "Pads are easy to change and you won't get so tired out from turning." The perineal area can also be padded unless the patient objects to the diapering concept. Short gowns or pajama tops will be less likely to become soiled with urine. Special attention should be given to the patient's general appearance to preserve or foster a positive body image.

If the patient's condition permits, a schedule can be worked out so that every two hours he can be helped to the toilet or commode or offered the bedpan. Giving the patient the opportunity to void 30 minutes to an hour after drinking fluids is another routine. Fluids might be restricted two hours before bedtime. Keeping a record of when or how often voiding occurs is another way to work out such a schedule. Unfortunately, bladder training takes time and many older patients are not in the hospital long enough for the nurse to record any success. The same suggestions might be valid for a bladder training program at home. The benefits of Kegel's exercises for women to help tone the muscles used in voiding are controversial. The woman is taught to contract the muscles as if trying to stop urinating and then relax them—this is repeated 10 to 15 times daily. However, many incontinent elderly people are confused and bladder training or bowel training is impossible.

Respiratory System: Nursing Responsibilities

Any developing chest pain or signs of respiratory distress such as shortness of breath or a cough, especially in the patient who is relatively immobile, must be reported to the physician immediately. Pulmonary embolism is a serious threat in older immobilized patients.

Deep breathing and coughing should be encouraged every four hours for the elderly patient who spends most of the day in bed or sitting in a chair. Age-related changes in the lungs make hard work out of coughing up secretions. If respiratory therapy has been ordered, the nurse should plan routines so that the patient has time to rest before attempting independently to use an incentive spirometer to promote lung expansion, or before having an intermittent positive pressure breathing (IPPB) treatment. Shortness of breath and dyspnea must always be noted. The kind and amount of sputum that is expectorated at any time should be documented.

Antiembolism Stockings

Since venous stasis is dangerous in immobilized older patients, antiembolism stockings are commonly ordered as a preventive measure. These stockings come in knee-high and full-length sizes. The nurse must remember two important points: knee-high stockings can be so high as to put pressure on the popliteal space or so tight as to *contribute to* venous stasis, and long stockings can roll like garters, also impairing circulation. All antiembolism stockings should be removed once every shift and the legs should be inspected for perspiration and redness. The legs must be dried thoroughly after the bath and before the stockings are reapplied at any time. The nurse may need to leave the stockings off for a period of time if the skin becomes irritated or the patient complains that the stockings are too hot. The condition of the patient's legs dictates how often the stockings should be checked and readjusted.

Getting the Patient Moving

Transfer

There is no *best* procedure for getting older patients out of bed. Helpless patients are more efficiently lifted by transfer boards, lifting sheets, and Hoyer lifts. From one to three people may be required when a patient needs assistance. There are some rules that must be followed:

- Remember an older person may have a fear of falling. Be patient and gentle; use extra help the first time the person is being assisted in getting out of bed.
- Encourage the older patient to use the trapeze if the bed has an overhead frame. Having some control over one's movements promotes safety.

- When getting the older patient into a wheelchair or geriatric chair, be sure it is locked into position.
- Bring the patient all the way to the edge of the bed.
- If the patient is tall, raise the entire bed so he does not have to bend forward but can more or less slide off the edge.
- Remember that older people have diminished sensations of pressure. Be sure an older patient can feel his feet on the floor before you move him.
- A transfer belt around the waist provides the security of having something extra to hold on to if necessary (Fig. 9–6).
- The patient should be wearing slippers or shoes with nonskid soles.
- The patient should be encouraged to take deep breaths before being helped out of bed.
- When lifting or helping the patient off the bed, stand as close to him as possible. Place your knees against his knees or your toes against his toes as you lift. Your arms should be around the waist, firmly grasping the belt, or up and under the arms and over the shoulders.
- The older patient can not sit in *any* chair for longer than two hours without a shift in position.

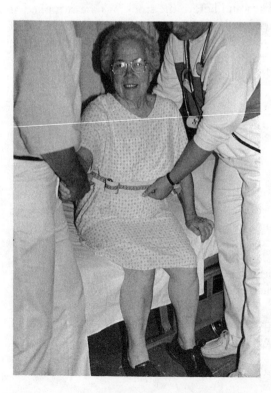

Figure 9–6. When getting an older patient out of bed, have her use shoes with nonskid soles, a safety belt, and help her to the edge of the bed.

Ambulation: Using Assistive Devices

In the hospital, many older patients walk with canes or walkers. A physical therapist should instruct the patient who is in a rehabilitation program following surgery, injury, or stroke. Sometimes patients with weakness or dizziness have a cane or walker, which is ordered for security. In general, the nurse should know the following about assistive devices:

- The elbow(s) should be at a 25- to 30-degree angle when using any assistive device.
- The patient should always walk by putting one foot in front of the other (Fig. 9–7); the involved extremity, if there is one, should go forward first. Patients using assistive devices have a tendency to put one foot forward, bring the other foot next to it, stop and then repeat the process advancing in a step–stop pattern.
- The patient should be instructed to stand tall, look straight ahead, and not watch the feet.
- The patient should be taught never to lean on a walker when getting out of a chair.

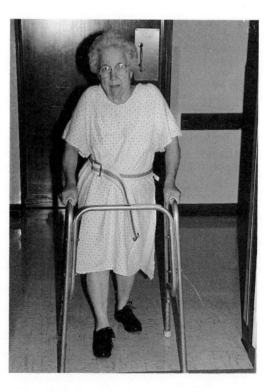

Figure 9–7. Using a walker, the patient is taught to look straight ahead and move by putting one foot in front of the other.

- The hand grips and tips of walkers and canes should be changed if they are worn smooth.

The nurse should observe the progress of older patients when they are ambulating so that she can reinforce therapy instructions and offer encouragement and praise.

Nutrition in the Hospitalized Patient

Factors in Eating

If the older person does not eat well, there are a number of factors to consider in addition to health problems and pain. There are age-related problems of sensory deficits and poor dentition and psychological factors that contribute to the poor eating habits of older people (see Chap. 7). In the hospital, older patients may not eat well because they are frightened or depressed. They may not like the hospital food or the hours at which meal trays are served. They may feel rushed and they may not have enough time to finish meals. Sitting up in bed to eat can be especially uncomfortable for them. Perhaps the patient on a general diet is not eating well because he had difficulty understanding or seeing the menu and did not want to ask for help; illiteracy may also be a problem. Besides its unappetizing appearance, pureed or soft food on a tray may be humiliating to the older patient, who feels that he is being treated like a "baby."

The plastic wrappings and covers on food, milk cartons, and tiny packets of salt, pepper, and sugar are difficult for older fingers to manipulate. When an older patient does not finish a meal, this may be part of the reason.

Older patients benefit from the one-on-one attention that is available from a hospital dietitian. The importance of proper nutrition to promote healing after surgery must be emphasized by the nurse, and a visit from the dietitian as soon as oral intake has been re-established will reinforce this point.

Tube Feedings

Tube feedings deliver a liquid diet directly into the stomach or small intestine when the patient is incapable of eating. The feeding may be intermittent or continuous. Indications for tube feedings include coma, dysphagia, surgery on the head or neck, and severe depression. The solution is ordered by the physician and obtained from the dietary department. Hospitals have standard policies and procedures for inserting feeding tubes and administering the solution. The following are general guidelines for preventing aspiration:

- Keep the head of the bed elevated during and at least 30 minutes after feedings.
- Discontinue the feeding if the patient needs to be supine for any reason or when there will be activity involving the chest.
- Check the residual in the stomach by aspirating at regular intervals until less than a specified amount is obtained. When residual remains over this amount, the physician must be notified.
- Check the position of the feeding tube in the nose and back of the throat and by *gently* aspirating stomach contents, as ordered. Initial placement of the tube should be confirmed by x-ray.

Other nursing responsibilities are as follows:

- Maintain intake and output.
- Weigh the patient as ordered.
- Flush the tube before and after giving medications.
- Remove the solution from the refrigerator about 30 minutes before hanging it to make sure it is room temperature. Cold solution will give the patient cramps and diarrhea.
- Take care of the patient's nose and mouth.
- Report prolonged or copious diarrhea, projectile vomiting, chronic constipation or fecal impactions, or weight loss.

Hyperalimentation

Hyperalimentation is the intravenous administration of nutrients into a central vein, ideally the superior vena cava. The term total parenteral nutrition, or TPN, is sometimes used instead of hyperalimentation. Patients who are unable to eat or to tolerate tube feedings may be candidates. The procedure must be done under strict aseptic technique to prevent infection. It is important to weigh the patient daily, maintain accurate intake and output, and watch for signs of infection. The urine is routinely checked for the presence of sugar, which indicates that the solution is running too fast for the body to metabolize the glucose. Careful observation of the total patient is required.

The Patient Receiving Intravenous Therapy

Often a patient who has intravenous fluids infusing will become restless or uncooperative because of the position of the arm. Positioning an upper

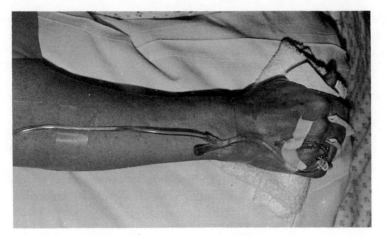

Figure 9–8. A hand with an IV should be flexed and supported, and it should have gauze between the fingers.

extremity applies to the patient with an I.V. If the needle is in the antecubital space, the arm is extended and this will eventually cause muscle strain and fatigue. Massaging the shoulder and moving the hand and wrist will provide temporary and partial relief. The fingers need room to breathe. If the I.V. needle is in the back of the hand, a light layer of tissue or gauze between the fingers with the fingers slightly flexed and supported by a rolled or folded washcloth will be comfortable (Fig. 9–8)

Tape should be applied firmly but it should not be tightly stretched across the skin, which might cause skin breakdown and edema. Needle sites must be inspected closely every hour for signs of infiltration because the older patient's skin is fragile.

Regular observations must also be made for side-effects of any medication administered by this route. Intake and output must be strictly maintained on patients who are getting intravenous fluids.

The Older Patient at Night

Two physiological facts about sleeping are as follows: One, keeping the patient warm will promote vasodilation and a good blood supply to wounds that may be healing. Two, a growth hormone is secreted during sleep that helps the body use protein, aiding in wound healing.

There is really no good sedative or tranquilizer for the elderly patient. In fact, a sleeping pill often causes agitation instead of restfulness. Making the patient comfortable and adapting to the patient's nighttime routine may be more beneficial (see Chap. 6).

Restricted positions such as those made necessary by surgical procedures, treatments, and intravenous therapy may make sleeping difficult. Anxieties and fears are magnified during the night, and pain may be more intense. These are other causes of insomnia in the hospitalized elderly:

- Unfamiliar surroundings
- Noise
- Hunger
- Too much caffeine
- Deprivation of tobacco when one has been a chronic user
- Nursing routines and observations
- Concern over getting to the bathroom "in time"

Sleep Apnea

Abnormal breathing during sleep is fairly common in older people, especially those with COPD. Sleep apnea—when breathing actually stops for more than ten seconds—can be observed in apparently normal individuals. When checking older patients at night, the nurse must be aware of this phenomenon. Noisy snoring and abnormal movements may also be present in these patients. Disorientation and headaches may occur in the morning, and the patient may be excessively drowsy during the day. There are more severe symptoms that can occur following repeated episodes of sleep apnea; therefore, the nurse must observe and document sleep patterns of the older patient.

The Confused Patient

Causes

In an older patient, confusion may be a response to any of a number of problems:

Disease in any system
Trauma
Medications
Malnutrition
Anemia
Hypoxia
Infection
Toxic substances
Lack of sleep
Disruption of familiar routines

Abnormal blood chemistry
Fluid and electrolyte imbalance
Pain
Overstimulation or understimulation

Remember that some confusion due to age-related changes is normal (see Chap. 6).

Nursing Implications

The nurse helps identify and correct causes of confusion and acts to protect the patient from injury and other problems. When the patient is confused, the dilemma for the nurse is not necessarily the confusion, but the agitation and lack of cooperation that goes with it. Thorough basic nursing care helps alleviate agitation by eliminating a number of potential causes of increased confusion, for example, deep breathing and moving the extremities increase circulation and blood supply to the brain. The following are other important guidelines for the nurse:

- Avoid startling the confused patient. For example, speak gently and pleasantly *as* you approach the bedside.
- Pay attention to complaints of hunger and thirst even if the patient has just eaten. Offer the patient a drink of juice or milk and a cracker if possible. To tell the patient he "can't be hungry" or "you just finished lunch" is to imply that he does not know what he is talking about. The same thing applies if the patient complains of being tired or in pain.
- Distract the patient who is showing signs of agitation. For example, say, "I like that new plant. Do you have plants at home?" or, "Do you like music?"
- Stop what you are doing whenever the patient is resisting all your efforts to provide care. Anything else is futile. Maybe it's time for more "TLC." Squeeze the patient's hand, stroke the arm. Perhaps say, "Rest a while."
- If the patient raises his voice, wait for an opportunity to speak and then do so in a soft tone.

Reality Orientation and Validation Therapy

Reality orientation is the process of gently correcting the patient who gives the wrong information, and trying to bring him back to the present. Here is an example:

Patient: "I am going to the store today."

Nurse: "You are in the hospital today, Mr. B."

Reality orientation may be most successful when used with the patient who has *periods* of confusion. Orientation to time and place may involve marked calendars or some kind of display board with information on it in big letters and numbers. Place clocks where the patient can see them as another orientation measure.

Validation therapy is communicating at the patient's level to help the patient cope with feelings rather than discuss facts. The nurse does not agree or disagree with what the patient is saying but asks questions and makes comments that will allow the patient to remember and to talk about subjects that have emotional meaning for him. As a result, the patient may be more peaceful and the nurse can sometimes learn about the purpose of the patient's behavior. Validation therapy may be more applicable when communicating with the patient who has dementia.

Drugs and the Older Patient

Age-related changes and chronic disease cause drugs in the elderly to be poorly absorbed, distributed, metabolized, and excreted. Drugs can adversely affect the patient's physiological, mental, emotional, and functional status. The rate of age-related decline in body organs and enzymes varies. Each older person responds to drugs in an individual manner. There are no standard doses. Symptoms of drug reactions can occur in any body system, and all drugs are potentially dangerous. There are important points to remember about drug administration in nursing older patients:

- All drugs must be collected on admission so the physician can check them against what will be ordered in the hospital.
- Because adverse reactions and possible drug interactions are so numerous, the nurse must review them when a new drug is ordered.
- The nurse should investigate all new symptoms because they are potentially drug related.
- Patients with serious kidney and liver dysfunctions, or CHF, are especially vulnerable to adverse drug reactions.
- Intramuscular injections should not be given in immobile muscles. If the patient is bedridden or confined to a wheelchair, injections should be given in the deltoid muscle where there is more movement and the blood flow is better.
- Older patients are more susceptible to the adverse effects of antibiotics, and they may respond more slowly to antibiotic therapy.

- Drugs used in the treatment of anxiety, depression and psychoses may aggravate the condition.
- Upon discharge from the hospital, the patient must be instructed in how to take all medications. Figure 9-9 is a sample discharge medication instruction sheet.

Drug Name	Drug Use	Tape Pill Down	Times	Special Instructions
Lasix 40 mg	Water pill		Take 1 pill twice daily 8 a.m. 4 p.m.	May change times. Take early morning and late afternoon so you aren't up to bathroom all night.
KCl 20 meq	Replaces potassium lost because of water pill.		Take 2 10 meq capsules twice daily. 8 a.m. 6 p.m.	Take with food or meals.
Lanoxin .25 mg	Strengthen and slow heart rate		Take 1 daily in a.m. 7 a.m.	Take before breakfast. Call doctor if nauseated or vomiting.
Ampicillin 500 mg	Antibiotic		Take 1 pill 4 times daily 7 a.m. 11 a.m. 4 p.m. 10 p.m.	On *empty* stomach.

ADDITIONAL COMMENTS: Green Bay and De Pere pharmacies will tape a sample of your pills on this sheet for you, upon request.

Other Areas: Please note that various brands of these drugs may appear of different color, size, or shape. You may wish to ask your local pharmacist to tape a sample of your pills on this sheet.

Figure 9-9. Medication instruction sheet. (Courtesy of Bellin Memorial Hospital, Green Bay, Wisconsin)

Special Needs of the Older Surgical Patient

Preoperative Considerations

An older person comes to the hospital for surgery with memories from other hospitalizations and other operations, if not his own, then those of families, friends, and neighbors. These memories, both good and bad, profoundly affect the patient's behavior. Although the nurse tends to view a surgical procedure as a positive event that will improve the quality of life, the older patient may have mixed feelings.

Preoperative fears may include fear of anesthesia. The patient may wonder if he will go to sleep and never wake up. Or a patient may dread spinal anesthesia for fear of paralysis. Back pain and stiffness also will contribute to a reluctance to undergo spinal anesthesia.

Preoperative instructions must be simple and based on what the patient wants to know. If the patient says, "It's all in God's hands," or "I don't want to know anything about it," the nurse must limit efforts to answering questions.

An older patient may be extremely self-conscious and fearful about being wheeled to surgery minus glasses, dentures, and hearing aid. A touch and some words of reassurance after transfer to the stretcher will help alleviate the anxiety of the patient who suddenly can't see well, hear well, or speak clearly. This patient will be more cooperative and less fearful in the operating room if the staff is made aware of his sensory deficits.

Postoperative Considerations

Cardiac arrest, postoperative hemorrhage and shock, thrombosis, pulmonary complications, and infections are threats to the elderly patient who has had a surgical procedure. Intravenous solutions must be monitored, and the nurse must be alert to complaints of chest pain, which may indicate cardiac overload. Deep breathing, coughing, and moving the extremities early in the postoperative period are imperative. Restlessness and confusion may be due to hypoxia, drugs, a full bladder, intravenous infiltration, or strain on an arthritic joint.

The older surgical patient is at high risk for postoperative infection because of these factors:

• Thin, dry skin, which will easily break down from irritation caused by dressings and tape

- Weak immune responses
- Nutritional deficiencies
- Lowered resistance because of restriction of oral intake in the pre-operative period
- Increased residual urine
- Ineffective cough
- Impaired circulation

Infection, other than wound infection, may be difficult to diagnose because the older patient may have only a slight temperature elevation. An additional factor that contributes to increased risk of wound infection in the elderly is that in moments of confusion an older patient often picks at a surgical dressing or at the incision itself.

The following measures prevent wound infection:

- Check dressings fequently (Fig. 9–10).
- Watch for redness and edema around the tape; if it occurs, loosen the tape and report this observation to the surgeon. Redness around the tape usually means redness under the tape.
- Reinforce and change dressings as necessary.
- Adhere strictly to aseptic technique when caring for wound drainage systems. Drainage containers should be emptied only when they are decompressed or full unless otherwise ordered.
- Encourage good nutrition and adequate fluids.

Remember that the uncooperative or combative postoperative patient may not know any other way to respond to the invasion of privacy during nursing routines. For best results, small doses of analgesics should be given *before* discomfort becomes severe.

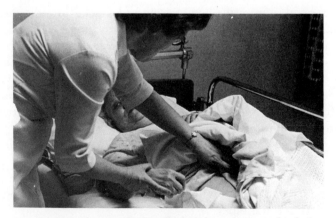

Figure 9–10. Frequent dressing checks help prevent wound infection.

The Elderly Surgical Outpatient

Brief and simple instructions on what to expect is essential in the care of the elderly person who is having outpatient surgery. This means what to expect in the hospital and what to expect at home (see the display, "What the Older Outpatient Needs to Know"). Written instruction sheets for all types of procedures may be provided by individual surgeons or by the hospital. Patients need specific information about what to do about postoperative bleeding, swelling, and pain and about the extent to which these postoperative conditions are normal. An older patient may tolerate more discomfort than he should or more bleeding than is safe simply because no one has told him that it is not normal, and he has learned to endure and expect problems (see the display, "Patient Information").

Psychological Considerations

The feelings of helplessness and dependency that develop when an older person is hospitalized are magnified by loss of identity, loss of control, and loss of privacy.

The patient is interviewed, undressed, examined, and put to bed, often in a hospital gown, in an unfamiliar room and he is identified by a nameband. Since the patient must adjust to certain routines as well as to the environment, the nurse must make every effort to individualize nursing care. Choices are important: the patient should be able to make some food choices and wear his own pajamas and robe. Whenever possible, ask questions in recognition of the patient's right to make choices:

(Text continues on p. 268.)

What the Older Outpatient Needs to Know:

- What is this test?
- What do I have to do to prepare for it?
- What can I eat the night before?
- Is it safe?
- Why *this* test—is it the best?
- What can I expect the day of the test?
- What if I have to cancel my appointment?
- Is it covered by Medicare (or my insurance)?
- When will I know the results?

Patient Information: Discharge Instructions and Care after Eye Surgery

Your operated eye will take approximately six to eight weeks to heal. To prevent any complications, it is important for you to understand and follow these instructions carefully.

Your vision may be somewhat blurry until the corrective lens in your glasses is changed, approximately six weeks after surgery.

DO NOT REMOVE EYE PATCH UNTIL _____

Protection of Your Eye

- Your operated eye should be protected at all times either by your glasses or a metal eye shield. The eye shield must be used while you are sleeping for six weeks following surgery.
- Do not get water or anything unclean into your eye.
- You may shower from the neck down.
- Avoid vigorous shaving and brushing teeth and hair. May wash hair gently after one week.
- Never wipe your eye with a soiled tissue or handkerchief.
- Do not rub your eye.

Activity

This is a general guideline. Check with your doctor about your individual case.

- While your eye is healing, avoid bending, stooping, or lifting anything heavy (*i.e.*, suitcases, groceries, or grandchildren).
- Refrain from sexual activity for two to three weeks.
- Avoid running, jumping, sudden jerky movements, or exerting yourself excessively at anything for six weeks.
- May go for walks and car rides.
- May swim after six weeks.
- May watch television and read if possible.
- For your own safety, please check with your doctor before driving an automobile.

Do Not Strain Your Eye

- Do not blow your nose too hard.
- Avoid coughing and sneezing. (You may want to give up pepper and powder.)
- Try not to become constipated and avoid straining heavily during a bowel movement.
- Do not squeeze your eyes shut.

continued

- Do not lie on your operated side. (Lie on your back or on your unoperated side.)

Call Your Doctor if You Have Any of the Following Signs or Symptoms

- Bleeding in your eye.
- A pus-like discharge from your eye.
- Sudden sharp pain in your eye that is not relieved by pain medication.
- Sudden change in your vision.
- Development of a cold or upper respiratory infection in which you must strain at coughing or blowing your nose.
- Sudden fever.

Medicines

- Wash hands thoroughly before eye care.
- The nurses in the Day Surgery Department will review with you or a family member how to administer your eye medication. Refer to "Preoperative Instructions: Instillation of eye drops."
- Be sure to bring your eye drops to each appointment with the doctor after surgery.
- Resume any medications you were taking from other doctors when you get home.

PUT _____ DROP(S) OF _____ IN THE OPERATED
EYE _____ TIMES A DAY.
PUT _____ DROP(S) OF _____ IN THE OPERATED
EYE _____ TIMES A DAY.
PUT _____ DROP(S) OF _____ IN THE OPERATED
EYE _____ TIMES A DAY.

Medications:

_____ Have prescription(s) filled at a pharmacy.
_____ Additional instructions: _____
_____

Next Appointment Time:

You should see _____ on _____
at _____ in his office.

(Courtesy of St. Mary's Hospital, Milwaukee, Wisconsin)

"Where would you like to walk?"
"Where would you like to sit today?"
"Where would you like me to take you in the wheelchair?"
"Shall I leave the door open? Blinds up?"

Showing respect for the patient as an individual helps preserve identity. Ask the patient, "What would you like me to call you?"

Positive comments on appearance and clothing along with encouragement in self-care increases the patient's sense of dignity and self-worth. Patients give nurses clues as to what is important to them. Here is an example:

Mrs. H, 69 years old, was hospitalized to have her diabetes controlled. She brought along a red wig and a makeup kit even though she was nauseated, vomiting, and quite weak. This should tell the nurse that Mrs. H is very conscious of the way she looks to others.

Many older patients are worried about finances and, in particular, what health costs will or will not be paid for by Medicare. The nurse should know which hospital staff member answers questions about Medicare and she should arrange for that person to talk to the patient.

Depression, as a sign of stress, is so common in older persons that one is tempted to dismiss it as a problem of aging and to concentrate efforts on "cheering up" the depressed person. The patient who appears sad, gloomy, or unusually quiet may need an opportunity to talk about general concerns or about particular procedures (see the display, "How to Ease the Stress of a Diagnostic Test").

The ways to initiate communication depend on the situation. The nurse might say to the patient, "Tell me about your day." A willing response on the part of the patient to questions of this nature opens the door for more specific questions. There are decisions that older patients must make that cause them great anxiety. For example, a 70-year-old man has coronary artery disease, and his kidneys are not functioning at an optimal level. He has been told that if he consents to bypass surgery, he has a 20% chance of not surviving the operation. If he does not have the operation, he has about one year to live.

Safety

Use of Restraints

Restraints of any kind should be used only as a last resort, that is, to protect the patient or someone else from injury. All restraints used on older patients must be made of soft material. The following are three warnings about the use of restraints:

How To Ease the Stress of a Diagnostic Test

Before

1. Teach the patient in simple language what is going to happen. For example, a CAT scan could be described in the following manner: "The technician will place you on a long table and you will be guided through a machine that is like a big doughnut. It will go around you and take x-rays."
2. Ask if the patient understands and has any questions. If patient is to be NPO, this must be clearly understood.
3. Be sure the patient is covered well, in wheelchair or on stretcher, and offer to send an extra blanket along to the testing department. Hallways, elevators, and waiting rooms are usually cool. Anxiety often brings "shivers."
4. In the department where the test will take place, be sure someone knows the patient is waiting. If the patient has a visual or hearing problem or any difficulty understanding directions, tell someone in the department.

After

1. Following a diagnostic test, older patients often experience dizziness or confusion due to stress or from being NPO. Watch for signs and give necessary assistance so the patient does not fall when getting back into bed.
2. Check B.P. and P.
3. If the patient has been NPO, offer juice, water, other appropriate fluid, or meal tray immediately.
4. Give medications that were withheld if this does not conflict with any medication schedule.
5. Ask the patient if he has any questions about the test and what happened during the test.

- Patients often become agitated and pull against their restraints, cutting off circulation.
- Restraints rub and dig into the skin and may cause skin breakdown.
- Restraints contribute to immobility.

Health care institutions have policies and procedures governing the use of restraints; generally, restraints should not be used without a physician's order.

Siderails

For the following reasons, siderails are a vital safety measure for older patients when they are in bed:

- Hospital beds are narrow, and a patient who is accustomed to a wider bed may fall out of bed when turning.
- Pain, anxiety, position, and medications can contribute to restlessness or disorientation, predisposing the patient to a fall.
- Hospital beds sometimes need to be maintained in the high position. Should the patient attempt to get up at night, he could fall while trying to get to a standing position.

Use of siderails may vary from place to place. In some health care institutions, a release form may be signed by the patient, which will permit the nurse to leave siderails down. Such information must be documented on the chart and noted on the care plan. The nurse must explain to the patient why siderails are necessary, and she should instruct him to use the call light when he wishes to get up.

Discharge Planning

Shortened hospital stays have increased the importance of early discharge planning to ensure continuity of care (see the display, "Review for the Elderly Diabetic"). In order to assess needs, the discharge planner makes contact with the older patient and with those who will be responsible for care at home. Input from the physician, nurses, therapists, and other professionals who have participated in the plan of care is required for this process. If comprehensive services are needed, a staff meeting will be scheduled to discuss plans, which will be attended by the health care team and by family members.

Primary considerations for the patient who is going home are the patient's actual capabilities, the environment and how it can be adapted, and available community resources:

- Will the patient need nursing care? What kind and how often?
- Will any deficits in vision, hearing, or mobility limit the patient's ability to learn or to care for himself?
- Is there a spouse or other elderly person living in the same house? If so, that person's needs must also be considered.
- Will housekeeping or shopping assistance be required?
- Does the patient have any financial, legal, psychological, or recreational needs?

Review for the Elderly Diabetic

The elderly diabetic may be admitted to the hospital for health problems other than diabetes. The nurse should review the patient's understanding of diabetes and the control program some time before discharge so that instruction can be offered in areas in which it is needed.

The nurse should ask these questions:

- Can you tell me how you would know if your blood sugar is too high? What should you do about it?
- When would it be too low and what would you take for it?
- Explain how you test your blood sugar.
- What pills do you take for diabetes? When do you take them? Tell me the side-effects.
- Explain how you fill a syringe with insulin. Do you need a magnifying glass or glasses to see it?
- Step by step, how do you give yourself insulin?
- Tell me what your meals might be for one day.
- What do you do about diet and your pill or insulin when you are feeling sick?
- How do you get exercise?
- Who takes care of your toenails?

The nurse should inspect the feet for the following:

- Toenails that are too short
- Irritation or scaly skin between the toes
- Bruises, open areas
- Check for a pedal pulse on top of the foot or below the inside ankle bone

CASE STUDY

Mrs. P is an 83-year-old female who was admitted to the hospital through the Emergency Room with shortness of breath, nausea, and vomiting. She has a medical history of valvular disease. Her condition was diagnosed as congestive heart failure and an upper respiratory infection. After four days, she was discharged to her daughter's home. She would be treated by medications and bedrest.

The discharge planning nurse and the patient's daughter have an in-depth discussion about what kind of care Mrs. P will need. The nurse refers Mrs. P's daughter to a local medical equipment supply company where she can rent a commode. Home health care will not be needed at this time, but the patient's daughter may eventually need respite care. The nurse provides the names and telephone numbers of two local agencies from which this resource is available.

Discharging a patient to a nursing home is an alternative that affects the whole family. The decision to place an older relative in a nursing home can precipitate mixed feelings of guilt, sorrow, and relief. Every circumstance is different and nothing is typical. Some transitions are made quickly and smoothly, and some take much time and energy.

CASE STUDIES: FROM A DISCHARGE PLANNER'S NOTES:

CASE #1—70-YEAR-OLD FEMALE. DIABETIC—AMPUTEE

Talked to the patient's son and daughter-in-law at great length about nursing home placement for their mother. The patient is eager to go to nursing home "A," an extended care facility (ECF), because many of her friends are there. Son is reluctant; he and his wife feel they ought to try and take care of the patient first. They have agreed to try placing the mother in an extended care facility, and if she isn't "perfectly happy," they will take her home.

CASE #2—85-YEAR-OLD MALE. CONFUSION, G.I. BLEEDING

1. This patient is well known to discharge planning from previous admissions, when arrangements were made per his wife's request for patient to enter nursing home "B". He also was agreeable, and then demanded to return home 24 hours later. Now his wife is requesting placement again.
2. Long talk with wife again. Concerned about her ability to care for patient at home due to her own deteriorating health status. "I made a mistake" taking him out of nursing home last time. Patient sleeps days at home and keeps wife up all night. Home care has been tried on several occasions but wife did not feel it too helpful. Additionally, patient's past needs have not been for skilled health care, therefore not covered by Medicare, and wife did not feel she could afford to pay for help.
3. Wife still ambivalent about ECF placement even though she verbalizes inability to provide adequate care. Couple has no children. Wife has two sisters in town: her support system. Wife needs to be encouraged to maintain her own health. Patient alert. Agrees to ECF now but no doubt will make wife take him home later.

Transfer forms that must be filled out when a patient is transferred to a nursing home vary according to institution, and they provide valuable information for care planning (Fig. 9–11).

The Nursing Home Resident

"Nursing home" is a generic term that is used to describe any institution that offers long-term health care, especially to elderly people. However, there are specific levels of care, and a facility may be licensed to provide one or more of these. Regardless of where nursing is practiced, the fundamentals of quality nursing are the same.

Characteristics of Nursing Home Care

"This is home," says a director of nursing, defining the basic characteristic of care. "While a resident is here he is home. We individualize the environment with his own possessions just as we individualize his care. Each resident has a nursing care plan."

The concept of being home means having access to barber, beautician, religious services, and social activities (Fig. 9–12). The nursing home resident also needs an opportunity to have privacy for intimate contact with a significant other.

The health care team focuses on the capabilities, not the limitations, of the resident and seeks to maintain and improve his level of function. On admission, the rehabilitation potential of a resident is identified, used in planning care, and continuously evaluated. A patient who has had orthopedic surgery may be transferred to the nursing home, and his rehabilitation potential might be stated as follows: "Good. Plan three weeks of physical therapy and then return home." A person with a brain tumor may have the following note on admission: "Rehabilitation potential poor. Plan long-term stay." Rehabilitation potential is based on physical and mental status, which can change.

Total health care needs of long-term residents, such as flu shots and dental care, must be considered. A geriatrician comments, "We don't cure the long-term resident. Most of them have some form of dementia. Our goal is to keep them happy and healthy."

In the nursing home setting, incontinence and constipation are common and ongoing problems. Residents who are accustomed to laxatives, suppositories, or enemas as needed may have to remain on their regimen to prevent constipation. Bran in the diet may or may not be effective. Warm drinks may stimulate peristalsis. The best alternative may be to provide the resident with privacy and comfort during defecation and to

Patient: _____ Date: _____

NURSING: Self-Care Status Check Func. Level		Indep.	Unable	Needs Assist.	Comments
Ambulation	Bed-Chair				
	Walking				
	Stairs				
	Wheelchair				
	Crutches				
	Walker				
	Cane				
Activities	Bathe self				
	Dress self				
	Feed self				
	Brush teeth				
	Shaving				
	Toilet				
	Commode				
	Bedpan/Urinal				

Incontinence: ☐ Bladder ☐ Bowel

Bowel & Bladder Program ☐ Yes ☐ No

Catheter: Type _____ Date last changed: _____

Vital Signs: T__ P__ R__ BP__

Weight   Height   Date

Check if Pertinent: Describe in patient care plan

DISABILITIES	BEHAVIOR	COMMUNICATION
__Amputation	__Oriented	__Can Write
__Paralysis	__Forgetful	__Talks
__Contracture	__Noisy	__Understands Speaking
__Decubitus	__Confused	__Understands English
__Ostomy	__Withdrawn	__Language Barrier
__Other	__Wanders	__Reads
_____	__Combative	__Nonverbal

IMPAIRMENTS   **APPLIANCES/PROSTHESIS**
Check "S" If sent; "N" If needed.

IMPAIRMENTS	APPLIANCES	PROSTHESIS
__Speech	__Cane	__Dentures
__Hearing	__Crutches	__Eye Glasses
__Vision	__Walker	__Hearing Aid
__Sensation	__Wheelchair	__Prosthesis (type)
__Other	__Other_____	

Comments:_____

Allergies:

Special prob./approaches rel. to administration of meds/treatments diet:

Skin/wound care:

Sleep/rest pattern including aids used:

Level of pt.'s understanding and/or motivation:

Teaching done or needed:
_____

R.N. Signature   Date   Work Phone

Social Information

Religion:_____

Marital Status: S__ M__ W__ D__ Sep.__

Information regarding pt.'s attitude, support system:

Short/long range plans to meet pt's needs:

Previously pt. lived: with family__ alone__ with friends__ nursing home__ other__

Discharge Planner   Date   Work Phone

Figure 9–11. Hospital Referral for Continuity of Patient Care. (Courtesy of Bellin Memorial Hospital, Green Bay, Wisconsin)

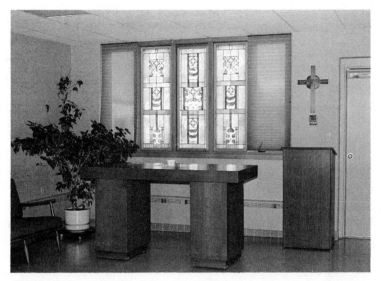

Figure 9–12. *A chapel may be at one end of the activity room in a nursing home.*

stay with routines the resident has worked out over the years. Depression, nervousness, sensory deficits, and tobacco or alcohol dependency are common long-term concerns that must be addressed according to the personality and condition of the individual resident.

Each level of nursing personnel must do a certain amount of assessment (Fig. 9–13). The registered nurse has daily contact with each

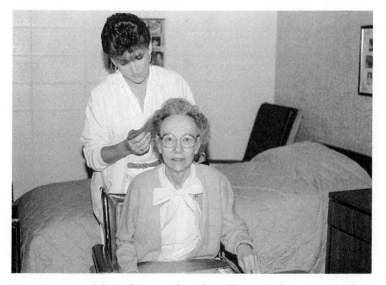

Figure 9–13. *While combing a resident's hair, the nursing home nurse is able to identify other needs.*

resident and makes assessments as changes occur in their status. In those facilities where the nursing assistants and licensed practical nurses do most of the hands-on care, there must be especially close communication and sharing of information because the observations of these team members are necessary and valuable.

Physicians make infrequent visits to their nursing home patients unless they have serious problems, so the physician depends on astute nursing assessment. The large number of medications most residents receive requires the nursing staff to be alert for adverse reactions and interactions. Residents often remain in a nursing home until they die, and those who care for them must be familiar with the signs of approaching death (see Chap 10).

The nursing home nurse is actively involved in the rehabilitation and daily life of the residents. Physical therapy may be a contracted or part-time service. Therefore, the nurse may be responsible for following through on rehabilitation goals for regular exercise and improved ambulation (Fig. 9–14). Residents and nurses get to know each other and may share social activities such as "pizza days" and parties on special occasions.

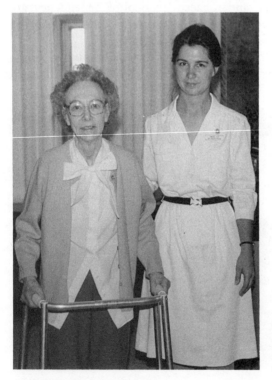

Figure 9–14. Walking a resident to the dining room, the nurse is working toward rehabilitation goals.

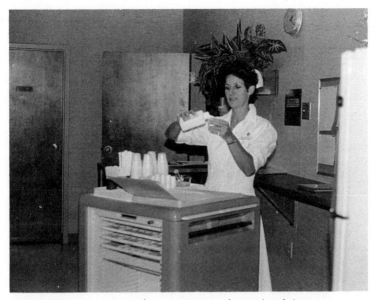

Figure 9–15. A nursing home nurse spends much of her time giving medications.

Daily Routines

Each nursing home resident has a care plan. Much of the nurse's time is spent in giving medications (see Fig. 9–15). Tub baths, showers, whirlpools, and bed baths are scheduled as needed, but daily bathing is uncommon. Taking blood pressures and giving decubiti care are usual routines.

Good handwashing techniques are continuously stressed to avoid infections and cross infections. Residents are taught and reminded to wash their hands after using toilet facilities and before meals. Residents are encouraged to eat in a dining room. Susceptibility to infections increases in residents with dehydration, diminished skin turgor, and bowel problems.

The nursing home resident at a custodial care level requires help with personal hygiene but no special treatments. Their medications are also given by nursing staff. Supervision may be the major nursing responsibility.

Nursing Home Dilemmas

The nurse must help the family remember why the older person is in the nursing home. This is the practical side of geriatric nursing, and it is often the source of dilemmas.

CASE STUDIES

Mrs. H is 82, obese, and slightly confused at times. She has two compression fractures in her vertebrae due to osteoporosis. She is in the nursing home because she can not care for herself due to back pain. Her obesity contributes to her discomfort, and she is on a weight reduction diet. On the third day after she was admitted, she began to beg for more snacks and more to eat. After two days of encouraging her to follow the diet, the nurse finally called the physician because the patient's nephew had threatened several times to do so. The doctor asked, "Well, what shall we do? Shall we do our job and keep her on a diet because it might help her back pain? Or let her eat what she wants because she might do it anyway?"

Mrs. T is 91 with Alzheimer's disease and a venous stasis ulcer on her right lower leg, which is clean but not healing. Although usually cheerful and cooperative, there are times when Mrs. T will not let the nurse near her to irrigate and dress the ulcer. In fact, she may throw a water pitcher. One day Mrs. T's daughter approaches the nurse, concerned that the ulcer isn't healing, and says, "It doesn't look like anyone is taking care of it." What should the nurse tell her?

Mr. D is another resident with Alzheimer's disease. His appetite is becoming progressively poorer, which is normal. Some of the nursing staff and some family members are now "thinking" perhaps Mr. D should have tube feedings. Should he? Will he leave the tube in place? In the long run, is this a "kind" or realistic approach to take?

These types of dilemmas have no easy solutions. What does quality of care mean, and what about the quality of life? The starting point for helping family members to make difficult and often heartbreaking decisions may be a discussion of what is actually happening to their older relative and what will make that person most comfortable. This approach may ultimately decrease frustration among the care-givers by allowing them to direct their energies toward realistic goals. This is difficult when one has cared for the same resident for weeks or months and has grown to "love" that person.

Reminiscence Therapy

Reminiscing or recalling long-forgotten facts, people, events, and feelings is a frequent pastime of older people. It is part of one's life review, and it helps the older person find a purpose for having lived; perhaps it makes it easier to face death. Remembering can be painful, but remembering can also ease the pain of an experience, and it can help one to understand the why and how of the experience. Resolving long-buried conflicts that arise in reminiscing and forgiving what one was determined never to forgive can bring a wonderful peace. A sense of completeness is an outcome of the process of remembering, reflecting, and putting together the pieces of one's life.

Group activities in nursing homes that promote reminiscence include asking questions about remembering, or holding classes on creative writing, drawing, or painting.

Ask residents to describe (or draw or paint) the following:

Your favorite birthday present
Your house
Your bedroom
A best friend
All the things of a certain season
A family member

Laughter, tears, and a wealth of words spill out during this kind of activity. Reminiscence therapy is beneficial for the residents, and it is an excellent way for the nurse to gain understanding of those older persons for whom she is responsible.

Pet Therapy

Nursing homes have policies about pets. Pets may be allowed in certain areas at specific times. For some older persons, a pet is a best friend, and contact with the pet will aid in reality orientation and relieve depression.

Intergenerational Activities

The nurse might investigate the possibility of having a high school class come for a Saturday night dance or a group of grade school children give a Christmas concert. These activities are enjoyed by all, and they promote understanding between age groups.

Dying and the Older Patient

A Review of Death and Dying

Elisabeth Kubler-Ross, whose work in the area of death and dying has become well known, identified five stages in the emotional process of dying and grieving. A dying person or the grieving family does not necessarily go through these stages *in order*, and they may not go through some of them at all. From her research, Kubler-Ross concluded that if a person is able to express the feelings associated with each of these stages, it may be easier for that person to accept the end of life.

Kubler-Ross defines the five stages as follows:

1. *Denial*—The person does not/can not accept that this is happening to him.
2. *Anger*—When a person *believes* he is dying, it is logical to be angry. This is also the time for blaming others and for finding fault with care and treatment.
3. *Bargaining*—This stage is best described by an example: "Please God, let me live and I promise I'll be a better person."
4. *Depression*—The finality of death is comprehended and the person realizes there are things he will never do again, or do at all, and that his days with family and friends are numbered. Regrets come easily to mind along with great sadness and deep concern for others.
5. *Acceptance*—In this stage, the person understands and accepts the fact that he is going to die. Often there is an attempt to take care of unfinished business and to help loved ones, who will be left behind, to cope with what is happening.

Dying in an Institution

Most elderly people die in hospitals or nursing homes because, for one reason or another, that is where *someone else* put them. In these settings, the dying elderly often feel lonely and isolated as the emphasis, especially in the hospital, is on keeping people alive. Personal feelings about death, feelings of inadequacy, and lack of knowledge about the needs of dying people may cause a nurse to avoid the elderly patient who is fearing death.

There is a tendency to keep the dying patient in a quiet, darkened room, alone, or curtained off from others, and to carry on conversations in whispers. Although it is extremely important to realize that some people *want* to be alone at this time, it is even more important to realize that every dying person is still an individual. He should be given the opportunity to tell or show the nurse what kind of attention he desires. The dying elderly person who wants to be part of the activities of living as long as possible may have a sense of being abandoned if he is left alone. Unrelieved pain adds to loneliness and fear.

It is permissible for the nurse to be emotionally involved with the dying patient. The truth is, if one works at keeping the dying person in touch with life, it is difficult *not* to become emotionally involved. The nurse keeps the dying person in touch with life through conversation and actions, by allowing color, sound, and light to remain in the environment, and by permitting visitors at any time.

In providing care for these patients, the nurse must help them to preserve energy for whatever it is they *want* to do, however they want to spend the time that is left. Offering the dying person choices is one way to do this: "When do you want a bath?" or "Would you rather not feed yourself? Shall I help you?" Energy is conserved when anxiety is relieved. Peace of mind is fuel for the body.

By attending to those things that show the dying elderly person that he is still a special individual, the nurse helps the patient to grow in self-esteem at this critical time. Appearance is important, along with cleanliness. The person who is dying needs to feel human by being listened to, touched, and respected.

No Code and Terminal Care Orders

When older patients are very ill or in life-threatening situations, the nurse must know what to do. Specific guidelines for documenting and carrying out no-code and terminal care orders are spelled out in policies and procedures of health care institutions. The nurse must be familiar with these guidelines. These guidelines include the following:

1. Definition of terms that may be used in orders:
   - No code—cardiopulmonary resuscitation (CPR) will not be initiated
   - DNR—do not resuscitate
   - DD—death with dignity
   - Terminal care order—an order whereby a patient will not be kept alive by extraordinary measures
2. The procedure for getting physician's orders will explain what must be discussed and written. These orders will be very specific. In the event that *no* orders are written, CPR is initiated as necessary, and extraordinary measures are used in maintaining life.

The Living Will

Elderly people who are sick enough to die may *want* to die, and yet they may allow others—physicians and family members—to make decisions for them. The "Living Will," a document that can be drawn up at any time, gives a person a chance to say how much he wants done to prolong life when that life is deteriorating (Fig. 9–16). The dying patient may change this will after it is made or ask for another to do so for him. The

SAMPLE*

Living will

DECLARATION

Declaration made this _____ day of _____ 199____,

I, _____,
being of sound mind, willfully and voluntarily make known my desires that my dying shall not be artificially prolonged under the circumstances set forth below, and do declare:

If at any time I should have an incurable injury, disease, or illness certified to be a terminal condition by two (2) physicians who have personally examined me, one of whom shall be my attending physician, and the physicians have determined that my death will occur whether or not life-sustaining procedures are utilized and where the application of life-sustaining procedures would serve only to artificially prolong the dying process, I direct that such procedures be withheld or withdrawn, and that I be permitted to die naturally with only the administration of medication or the performance of any medical procedure deemed necessary to provide me with comfort, care or to alleviate pain.

In the absence of my ability to give directions regarding the use of such life-sustaining procedures, it is my intention that this declaration shall be honored by my family and physician(s) as the final expression of my legal right to refuse medical or surgical treatment and accept the consequences from such refusal.

I understand the full import of this declaration and I am emotionally and mentally competent to make this declaration.

Signed _____

Address _____

I believe the declarant to be of sound mind. I did not sign the declarant's signature above for or at the direction of the declarant. I am at least 18-years of age and am not related to the declarant by blood or marriage, entitled to any portion of the estate of the declarant according to the laws of intestate succession of the _____ or under any will of the declarant or codicil thereto, or directly financially responsible for declarant's medical care. I am not the declarant's attending physician, an employee of the attending physician, or an employee of the health facility in which the declarant is a patient.

Witness _____

Address _____

Witness _____

Address _____

ss.:

Before me, the undersigned authority, on this _____ day of _____, 199____, personally appeared _____, _____, and _____, known to me to be the Declarant and the witnesses, respectively, whose names are signed to the foregoing instrument, and who, in the presence of each other, did subscribe their names to the attached Declaration (Living Will) on this date, and that said Declarant at the time of execution of said Declaration was over the age of eighteen (18) years and of sound mind.

[Seal]
My commission expires:

_____
Notary Public

*Check requirements of individual state statute.

Figure 9–16. *A sample living will, prepared for the US Senate Special Committee on Aging. (Reprinted with permission from Hoopes R: The Living Will, Modern Maturity, June/July 1988. Copyright 1988, American Association of Retired Persons)*

will is not always binding because a family member is able to act against it if the dying person is not capable of making decisions. There are also technical and ethical aspects from the physician's standpoint. The will's most useful purpose is to encourage the patient, the physician, and the family to talk seriously about decisions and responsibilities. This will eliminate some of the potential for feelings of guilt in the survivors and in the health care team after the patient has died. In many institutions, a policy about the Living Will can be found in the policies and procedures manual, and the forms are available in the nursing service office.

The issue is that the dying elderly person needs to know it is "okay" to die. The nurse must be knowledgeable about Living Wills, and she must be prepared to answer questions and to refer the family or the patient to the physician for appropriate input. States have laws relative to the use of Living Wills.

Hospice

Hospice is a program of care with a philosophy that focuses on helping the dying person to live a full life and to maintain control over treatment. The following are among the goals of a hospice program:

- Assist terminally ill patients in living the life of their choice until they die.
- Work with dying patients and their families in an atmosphere of realistic hope.
- Provide care that will meet the patient's needs for physical and psychological comfort.
- Allow patients to die naturally and with dignity.
- Support the families during the illness, at the time of death, and for a period of time in bereavement.

Home care is the primary component of today's hospice programs, and many of these programs are sponsored by home health agencies. Care is given by a hospice team of nurses, home health aids and helpers, companion sitters, and volunteers. So that the patient can die at home in peaceful and familiar surroundings, the family is instructed and supported in care-giving as each new need arises (see Chap. 10 for signs of approaching death for family use).

Although referrals are made by health care professionals, the patient, or the patient's family, the family physician is always contacted before care is begun. If the hospice patient agrees, he is admitted to the hospital when the physician feels there is a need for treatment of specific symptoms. The hospice team visits the patient and helps the nurse develop a care plan. Every effort is made to adjust hospital routines to the patient's needs and to make the patient's environment more home-like. Unlimited visiting privileges are extended to family and friends in accordance with the patient's wishes.

After the patient dies, bereavement support for the family is ongoing for about one year. Group therapy is available for adults and children (see the display, "The Hospice Person's Bill of Rights").

Legacies and Peaceful Death

An older person who is dying often wonders what his life was worth. Will he be remembered when he is gone? Who cares that he lived at all? The nurse should *listen* for clues that the patient is searching for answers to these kinds of questions. Words of regret and spoken memories are opportunities for the nurse to encourage some life review. Help the dying older patient discover the legacies he has left for others. What did he do that no one else could do in quite the same way? What is his claim to immortality? Although legacies are often material things, like money or treasured possessions, what one has shared with others to help them grow in their own lives is also a legacy. For the teacher, the nurse, or the creative artist, this kind of legacy is obvious. However, the uniqueness of each person means that his or her life had special meaning. The nurse can give reassurance about the special meaning of each person's life.

Does this make dying easier for the patient? Maybe. Perhaps acceptance of death is related to how one has accepted life and what one believes death is all about. The thought of death as a release from suffering may be comforting. Spiritual and religious beliefs may condition one for the moment of death. "Just because I'm old doesn't mean I've accepted death more than the young," is the comment of a very old lady. In dying, as in living, there is no such thing as an "average" old person.

Summary

Initial assessment and ongoing observations are essential to caring for the sick older person. The nurse looks at the total person during routine care, beginning with how that patient slept during the night. A head-to-toe inspection during the bath and assessment of body functioning are necessary. All complaints must be investigated. The patient who has difficulty in swallowing and speaking must have special care to maintain nutrition

The Hospice Person's Bill of Rights

I have the right to be treated as a living human being until I die.

I have the right to maintain a sense of hopefulness however changing its focus may be.

I have the right to be cared for by those who can maintain a sense of hopefulness, however changing this might be.

I have the right to express my feelings and emotions about my approaching death in my own way.

I have the right to participate in decisions concerning my care.

I have the right to expect continuing medical and nursing attention even though "cure" goals must be changed to "comfort" goals.

I have the right not to die alone.

I have the right to be free from pain.

I have the right to have my questions answered honestly.

I have the right not to be deceived.

I have the right to die in peace and dignity.

I have the right to retain my individuality and not be judged for my decisions which may be contrary to beliefs of others.

I have the right to discuss and enlarge my religious and/or spiritual experiences, whatever these may mean to others.

I have the right to expect that the sanctity of the human body will be respected after death.

I have the right to be cared for by caring, sensitive, knowledgeable people who will attempt to understand my needs and will be able to gain some satisfaction in helping me face death.

This Bill of Rights was created at a workshop on "The Terminally Ill Patient and the Helping Person" in Lansing, Michigan, sponsored by the Southwestern Michigan Inservice Education Council and conducted by Amelia J. Barbus, Associate Professor of Nursing, Wayne State University, Detroit.

and to identify needs. Because many older persons have vision and hearing deficits, the nurse must consider these possibilities. Hearing aids are common, and they need proper handling. Positioning a patient properly promotes comfort and cooperation. The patient's bowel and bladder habits must be known in order to prevent problems such as constipation and urinary incontinence.

Transfer and ambulation of older patients requires observation of general rules to insure safety. Alternative methods of nutrition include tube feedings, hyperalimentation, and intravenous feedings. Hospital policy dictates rules for care. Sleep apnea, insomnia, and wakefulness are fairly common, and they require the nurse to make vigilant observations of older patients at night. Reality orientation and validation therapy, frequently used in nursing homes, may help in communicating with confused persons. The older surgical patient needs care to prevent problems of mobility, and detailed instructions on procedures and routines. Comprehensive discharge planning must begin early. The basic difference in the care of older persons in nursing homes is that they are residents. Care plans reflect concern with daily routines and rehabilitation potential.

In caring for the older patient who is dying, the nurse should be aware that because one is old he is not necessarily ready to die. Providing comfort and allowing the patient to have the activity he desires should be nursing goals. The nurse must be knowledgeable about possible ethical and legal complications.

Activities

1. Ask an older relative the following questions:
   a. Has he ever been in a hospital?
   b. What kind of contact has he had with nurses?
   c. What would his feelings be if he had to be admitted to the hospital tomorrow with a broken leg?
2. What questions would you ask and what observations would you make if you were admitting the following patient:
   An 81-year-old woman is brought in by the rescue squad, accompanied by a neighbor who said he "found her lying on her kitchen floor." She has been put to bed and is conscious and crying.
3. Give examples in which proper positioning can alleviate or prevent pain in older patients.
4. Give a detailed description of presenting problems during tube feeding.

5. How would you respond to an older man who is scheduled for surgery and tells you he does not want spinal anesthesia?
6. Discuss what you would do for the older patient who tells you she "always gets constipated in the hospital."
7. Make a list of drugs commonly administered to older patients and the side-effects of these drugs.
8. Plan an intergenerational activity that you could sponsor in a local nursing home.
9. List four specific comfort measures for an older patient who is dying.
10. Talk to a terminally ill patient who is aware of his diagnosis. Determine what stage of dying he is in.
11. Complete the diabetic review with an older diabetic patient (see the display, "Review for the Elderly Diabetic," in this chapter).

Bibliography

Birchenall J, Streight M: Care of the Older Adult, 2nd ed. Philadelphia, JB Lippincott, 1982

Blakeslee J: Untie the elderly. Am J Nurs 88:833–834, 1988

Bowers A, Thompson J: Clinical Manual of Health Assessment. St. Louis, CV Mosby, 1984

Brock A: How do the aged cope with surgery? Today's OR Nurse 6:16, 20–25, 1984

Burgess W: Community Health Nursing: Philosophy, Process, and Practice. Norwalk, CT: Appleton Century Crofts, 1983

Burkle N: Inadvertent hypothermia. J Gerontol Nurs 14:26–30, 1988

Burnside I: Nursing and the Aged: A Self-Care Approach, 3rd ed. New York, McGraw-Hill, 1988

Carnevali D, Patrick M (eds): Nursing Management for the Elderly, 2nd ed. Philadelphia, JB Lippincott, 1986

Dellefield M: Caring for the elderly patient with cancer. Oncol Nurs Forum 13:19–27, 1986

Duescher N: Pressure sore management. Bellin Hospital, Green Bay, WI, 1988

Ebersole P, Hess P: Toward Healthy Aging: Human Needs and Nursing Response, 2nd ed. St. Louis, CV Mosby, 1985

Fulmer J: Lessons from a nursing home. Am J Nurs 87:332–333, 1987

Gaudine A: Not another fractured hip. Can Nurse 82:25–29, 1986

Gray-Vickrey M: Color them special: A sensible, sensitive guide to caring for elderly patients. Nursing 17:59–62, 1987

Griffin M: In the mind's eye . . . value of imagery. Am J Nurs 86:804–806, 1986

Lawson P, Strauch P, Best C (eds): Helping Geriatric Patients Nursing Photobook. Nursing 82 Books. Springhouse, Intermed. Communications, 1982

Huey F: What teaching nursing homes are teaching us. Am J Nurs 85:678–683, 1985

Jackson M: High-risk surgical patients (CEU exam questions). J Gerontol Nurs 14:8–15, 40–42, 1988

Jacobs L, Fontana R, Albert D: Is that geriatric really ready to go home? RN 48:40–42, 1985

Jacobs L, Fontana R, Albert D: RN master care plan: When the geriatric patient goes home. RN 48:43, 1985

Jones G: Validation therapy: A companion to reality orientation. Can Nurse 81:20–23, 1985

Kreulter P: Nutrition in Perspective. Englewood Cliffs, Prentice-Hall, 1980

Latz P, Wyble J: Elderly patients: Perioperative nursing implications. AORN J 46:238–252, 1987

Liddel D: An in-depth look at osteoporosis. Orthop Nurs 4:23–27, 1985

Maas M: Management of patients with Alzheimer's disease in long-term care facilities. Nurs Clin North Am 23:57–68, 1988

Malcom JD: Battle cry for Mr. MacDonald . . . to help a dependent patient . . . try capitalizing on his past. Nursing 15:44–46, 1985

McCormick K, Sheve A, Leahy E: Nursing management of urinary incontinence in geriatric inpatients. Nurs Clin North Am 23:231–262, 1988

Moore S: Stepping stones . . . senile dementia (case study). Nurs Times 81:41–44, 1985

Morton I, Bleathman C: Reality orientation: Does it matter whether it's Tuesday or Friday? Nurs Times 84:25–27, 1988

Patrick M et al: Medical–Surgical Nursing: Pathophysiological Concepts. Philadelphia, JB Lippincott, 1986

Pritchard V: Geriatric infections: Skin and soft tissue. RN 51(6):60–64, 1988

Pritchard V: Geriatric infections: The urinary tract. RN, 51(5):36–38, 1988

Pritchard V: Preventing and treating geriatric infections. RN 51(3):36–38, 1988

Ramsey R: Adjusting drug dosages for critically ill elderly patients. Nursing 18:47–49, 1988

Ratcliffe J: Worth a try. Nurs Times 84:29–30, 1988

Rosdahl C: Textbook of Basic Nursing, 4th ed. Philadelphia, JB Lippincott, 1985

Ross M: When sleep won't come: Helping our elderly clients. Can Nurse 82:14–18, 1986

Santo-Novak D: Seven keys to assessing the elderly. Nursing 18:60–63, 1988

Schulman B, Acquaviva T: Falls in the elderly. Nurse Pract 12:30–37, 1987

Spradley B: Community Health Nursing: Concepts and Practice, 2nd ed. Boston, Little, Brown and Co, 1985

Vickrey M: Color them special. Nursing 17:59–62, 1987

Warner D: Walking to better health. Am J Nurs 88:64–66, 1988

Westfall L, Pavlis R: Why the elderly are so vulnerable to drug reactions. RN 50:39–43, 1987

Williams L: Alzheimer's: The need for caring. J Gerontol Nurs 12:20–28, 1986

Worstall J: Caring for Kathleen. Nurs Times 83:28–30, 1987

Yurick A, Spier B, Robb S: The Aged Person and the Nursing Process, 2nd ed. Norwalk, CT: Appleton Century Crofts, 1984

10

Community Resources
for Care

Learning Objectives

When you complete this chapter, you should be able to:

1. Make general suggestions on locating community resources for elderly people at home.
2. Describe how to identify home care needs.
3. List examples of community resources.
4. Differentiate among these forms of care:
   a. Residential care facility
   b. Adult day care
   c. Respite care
   d. Home health care
5. Discuss these aspects of home health care:
   a. Advantages
   b. Levels
   c. Goals
   d. Assessment factors
   e. Special characteristics
6. Explain the procedure in selecting a nursing home.

When community resources are accessible, living with dignity and security can be a reality for an older person, regardless of his or her level of dependency. The spectrum of needs ranges from the need for transportation to the physician's office to the need for skilled nursing care. The nurse must understand what community resources are, how to locate and utilize them, and how to assist older people and their families to do the same.

For most older persons, living at home and selecting from a wide range of community services is the most desirable option. Others may prefer a retirement home that offers continuing care. One would hope that the older person who is recovering from illness, undergoing rehabilitation, and adjusting to dependency has access to community resources that will allow him to continue living at home (see Chap. 9).

With the help of relatives, friends, and professionals, an aging person who is homebound can benefit from a variety of services. In all cases, the emphasis is on meeting physical and psychological needs in a cost-effective manner. Long-term care needs can be costly.

Partnership among care-givers in the home and community agencies or individuals is the key to successful interdependent living for the aging person. For example, the home health nurse and the daughter who is caring for an ailing elderly mother confer about routines before they are begun, and they regularly evaluate results together. Home health care agencies, which provide different levels of care, are a growing segment of the health care industry. They offer excellent opportunities for the nurse with gerontological nursing skills.

General Information

Factors in Finding Care

The size of the community is one factor that determines the availability of local resources for the care of aging people who are ill and dependent. In any community, churches and libraries are potential sources of information about where to seek help. Crisis intervention centers, the health department, United Way, and social service agencies are other starting points. On the state level, there are Area Agencies on Aging (AAA) that are responsible for planning, coordinating, and funding many programs. These area offices have listings of resources. A Social Security Administration office can offer suggestions about whom to contact for help.

State laws influence the type and availability of programs and services. The increasing numbers of older people has led to more federal legislation addressing the problems of aging citizens. The 1988 Older Americans Act authorized several new programs, including more home care services to the frail elderly and more state grants for special needs. New outreach programs will help find those people who need and qualify for some federal assistance but are unable to apply for it or unaware that it is available.

Identifying Needs

The older person must evaluate his present living environment, daily functioning, and financial situation before choosing community resources for long-term care. Although the older person will often rely on relatives for assistance, he should make his own decisions whenever possible. A local social service agency can be helpful in providing professional assessment. Upon discharge from a health care facility or when seeking assistance to remain at home, the patient should be prepared to address these questions:

- Am I able to handle my personal needs?
- Can I run my own errands?
- Is transportation available when I need it?
- Do I have problems getting around my home?
- Do I need help with homemaking?
- Am I in need of any legal assistance?
- How about my finances? Can I pay my own bills?
- Do I feel safe in this neighborhood?
- How much help do I need? Full time? Part time?
- Do I feel like I need more social activity?

An older person should decide for himself which services are appropriate for his needs (Fig. 10–1).

Resources for Independent Living

Transportation

Contact the American Red Cross when checking into the availability of transportation. They may offer transportation for elderly people at a minimal cost. The Area Agency on Aging may offer assistance to older people who live in rural areas or even issue I.D. cards good for discounts on bus or taxi fares.

County social service departments are a potential resource. Transportation systems, such as vans that carry wheelchairs, may be available. Fees

SPECTRUM OF LONG-TERM CARE SERVICES
Do you need assistance with these activities?

	Little or No Assistance	Moderate Assistance	Cannot Perform without Assistance
Home	▓		
House Sharing	▓		
Home with — Chore Services — Senior Center — Nutrition Services	▓	▓	
Continuing-care Community	▓	▓	
Congregate Housing	▓	▓	
Home with — Delivered Meals — Homemaker • Home Health Aide • Board & Care Home • Telephone Reassurance • Visiting		▓	▓
Home with — Adult Day Care		▓	▓
Home with — Home Care — Respite Care			▓
Continuing-care Community (Nursing Care)			▓
Nursing Home			▓

Figure 10–1. The older person should decide how much assistance he needs with the following activities: housework, transportation, managing money, taking medication, eating, dressing, bathing and toileting. (Reprinted with permission from Modern Maturity. Copyright 1988, American Association of Retired Persons)

may be eligible for reimbursement under Medicare or Title XIX (see Chap 1).

Senior Centers

An array of community services is offered through multipurpose senior centers supported under the Older Americans Act. These places offer classes, sponsor bus trips, dances, and card parties, serve hot meals, have outreach programs, and are treasuries of helpful information (Fig. 10–2). A senior center is a place where older citizens can meet people, make new friends, and enjoy companionship.

Legal Assistance

Legal assistance may be necessary in matters of property transfer, rights under Medicare, interpreting insurance, drawing up a will, and deciding on a guardianship or power of attorney. Legal services agencies under the Older Americans project provide assistance to low-income elderly and even make special arrangements to see those people who cannot come to an office. An office on aging may offer legal advocacy and information on a variety of issues including consumer complaints and protective services. The American Civil Liberties Union and the local public defender's office may be sources of information at little or no cost.

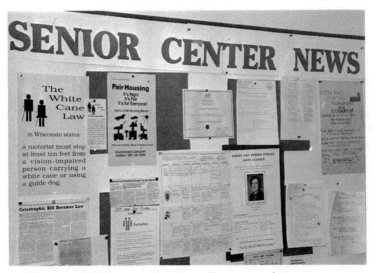

Figure 10–2. Multipurpose senior centers offer an array of community services.

294 Nursing Care of the Older Person

Financial Advice

Older people must be made aware that the Social Security office is the best place to get information about Social Security, no matter what they have read or heard. This office also has facts about retirement and survivor and disability insurance, as well as Supplemental Security Income. The State Department of Revenue will help with taxes and tax questions. Senior centers may have volunteers available on a scheduled basis to help older people with various tax forms.

Medicare Assistance

A legal services agency will help older people to remain updated on Medicare and interpret their rights. A hospital business or insurance office can provide assistance with the following:

- Submitting Medicare and supplemental insurance claims
- Reading and interpreting bills for medical services
- Filing a Medicare claims appeal
- Understanding explanations of benefits.

Reassurance Programs

A hospital may have a personal emergency response system designed to help the elderly person stay at home. A small electronic unit is carried by the older person at all times. Pressing a button alerts the hospital or an emergency telephone number that help is needed. The hospital also makes regular contact with the person who is wearing this kind of unit. This communication system can be established between family members and the older person by programming the unit with telephone numbers of those family members. Information about a personal response system can be obtained through the telephone company.

Senior citizen "hot lines" or telephone reassurance programs may be services of volunteer centers or senior centers. Hot lines are information centers, while a reassurance program usually involves another older person who makes calls regularly just to talk or to offer emotional support.

Protective Services

Abuse of the elderly is an issue in today's world (see Chap. 1). Social service departments commonly offer assistance to elderly people who have been abused or who are at risk. Even when relatives are loving and kind, an older person who is living alone will feel safer knowing that there are community agencies concerned about his or her safety.

Medical Equipment

Hospital supply companies may sell equipment to individuals for home use. They are listed in telephone books under "Home Health Care Supplies" and "Hospital Equipment and Supplies." Some pharmacies sell or rent home health care supplies (Fig. 10–3). The Veterans of Foreign Wars is a source of hospital beds, wheelchairs, and walkers, and one does not need to be a veteran to be eligible for assistance.

Counseling

A cleric is an appropriate person to ask about qualified counseling services in any community. Family service or social service agencies are also excellent contacts.

Meal Programs

Meals on Wheels programs assure delivery of one nutritious, hot meal daily to elderly people who are homebound. In large communities, there will be other mobile meal programs sponsored by hospitals and churches. Social service agencies, the local health department, the Visiting Nurses' Association (VNA) or a church could have telephone numbers of meal programs.

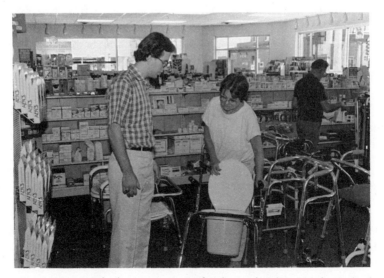

Figure 10–3. Medical equipment can often be purchased or rented at a local drugstore.

Companionship

Programs are available under area agencies or social service agencies to match older people with part-time or full-time companions. The Salvation Army has a visiting service.

Household Chores and Home Maintenance

An agency for the aged probably has a list of persons who will provide home care or maintenance services at a reasonable cost. Help around the home may also be available through social services. A state Job Service is another resource. Household help can be located through, and in conjunction with, home health care agencies.

Handicapped Parking

A permit to park in designated parking spaces will be issued by the State Department of Transportation to an elderly person with limited mobility who uses a cane, walker, or wheelchair. A physician's order is necessary. These permits can be placed on the dashboard of any vehicle the elderly person is riding in or driving.

Miscellaneous Resources

The Veterans Administration has services and information available for veterans and their dependents. Many older people may not be aware of this resource, although many are eligible for these benefits.

The telephone company and public utilities may be resources because they frequently offer special services to older people. For instance, a public services corporation may do a "house check" and suggest ways to conserve energy.

Older people should know that the local police department will give them tips on protecting themselves from crime in a variety of ways, from detecting fraud to making a home or apartment burglarproof.

Emergency Assistance

Social service, welfare departments, and churches can be called on by those older people in need of emergency help such as getting food, clothing, shelter, or medical assistance. The Salvation Army offers a wide range of helpful services to all kinds of people and in an emergency is an excellent resource.

Support Groups

Crisis intervention centers, hospitals, community service agencies, the United Way, and the American Red Cross are potential sources of information about support groups. There may be support groups for victims of chronic pulmonary obstructive disease, cardiomyopathy, diabetes, arthritis, impotence, cancer, and Alzheimer's disease. A support group functions to help the affected person and his family cope with problems and feelings and share experiences. Other goals of a support group can be educating the public, supporting research to find cures, and influencing pertinent legislation. A growing national association of special significance to the elderly and their care-givers is the Alzheimer's disease and Related Disorders Association, Inc. Contact them by writing to the following address or phoning the "800" number:

> Alzheimer's Disease and Related
> Disorders Association, Inc.
> 70 E. Lake Street
> Chicago, IL 60601-5997
> 1-800-621-0379

This association and its affiliates disseminate a wealth of information about the disease and assist in establishing day care programs for the afflicted and support groups for family members.

Residential Care Facilities

Services vary in residential care facilities. They may include a room, meals, utilities, laundry, and housekeeping as a "room and board" arrangement. Residents eat their meals together. In facilities with small apartments that include kitchens, there may still be a central dining room. Some degree of personal assistance and nursing care or supervision is also provided. A professional staff would include a registered nurse, nutritionist, social worker, and recreational specialist. There may be a physician available at regularly scheduled times.

The older person and his family should be advised that standards vary widely in these places because most of them are privately owned and operated. Although the facility may be regulated by fire, safety, zoning, and housing regulations, it may not have had to follow a specific licensing procedure. There are some useful suggestions to help a person select a suitable place:

- Visit the place under consideration, meet the administrator, and request a tour.
- Note the cleanliness and safety features and ask about security.

- Try to visit a number of the residents to determine if you will want them for neighbors. Ask them how they like the residence.
- Participate in a meal or social activity or both.
- Get information about any special services you might require.
- Check credentials of staff members.

Rehabilitation Services

Physical therapy, occupational therapy, and speech therapy are often provided in rehabilitation centers within a community. Private agencies also offer these services. The older person or someone responsible for his finances must know when a physician's prescription is required for therapy and who will pay the bill.

Adult Day Care and Respite Care

Older persons who need assistance, but not 24 hours a day, are good candidates for adult day care centers. These persons usually live with, or under the close supervision of, a family member who needs the relief that adult day care centers offer by taking temporary care of their aging relative. Adult day care emphasizes social activities and some rehabilitation. Hot meals, snacks, and assistance with medications are aspects of daily care. Showers and shampoos may be part of a weekly plan.

Respite care is temporary relief (overnight or for a short vacation) for the family care giver. This is sometimes a function of adult day care centers. Social service departments may have listings of adult sitters who will come to the home for respite care. Programs under the Older Americans Act provide both day care and respite care. Some respite care services originate in churches, synagogues, home health care agencies, and volunteer agencies.

The Veterans Administration has set up a number of free day care programs for veterans with long-term, disabling illnesses such as strokes or Alzheimer's disease. Where a health care team of physician, nurse, nutritionist, and therapists is available, the cost has been kept low. Poetry groups, reminiscence groups, and classes in ceramics, woodworking, singing, and exercise are the usual kinds of activities. A weekly visit from a chaplain is a feature of the Veterans Administration programs in many locations.

Home Health Care

Home health care is assistance in meeting health care needs in the home. The range of services is broad and includes skilled nursing, physical therapy, occupational therapy, speech therapy, personal care, housekeeping, companionship, and hospice care. The concept of home health care has been developed by community agencies such as local health departments or visiting nurses' associations, by independent agencies that employ some health care personnel and contract for other services from available providers, and by hospitals that set up their own agencies.

Home health care agencies make referrals to other community resources and work in close cooperation with hospitals and the medical community to assure that daily needs are met. As a consumer, the person receiving home care services has certain rights (see the display, "A Home Care Bill of Rights").

Reimbursement for home health care services comes from diverse sources; Medicare and Medicaid are the most common sources for older people. Private insurance companies and the Veterans Administration provide some payments. Funds allocated by the Older Americans Act may cover some home care costs. Individual communities may have other resources for those in need. For any kind of coverage, there are strict eligibility requirements that are subject to frequent change. An agency with Medicare certification is the logical choice for the older person who has complex health care needs.

Private insurance coverage varies from policy to policy and it is often vaguely described. An older person should be advised to submit claims even when reimbursement seems doubtful because each circumstance is unique.

Advantages of Home Health Care

Although not all medical problems can be treated at home, older persons who have long-term illnesses seem to fare better in their own environment. Many surgeons believe that postoperative ambulation increases in familiar surroundings, so wounds heal more rapidly. Psychologically, older people who can remain at home for health care have a greater sense of well-being because they know they have a resource available to them 24 hours a day while they are still in control of their own care. With adequate instructions, resources, and support, family members can successfully care for the terminally ill older relative in the home. Finally, the cost of quality home health care can be significantly less than the cost of comparable care in a hospital or nursing home.

Levels of Home Health Nursing Care

There are four levels of nursing care in home health. The registered nurse makes the initial visit, does the assessment, confers with the physician,

Home Care Bill of Rights

The National HomeCaring Council and the Council of Better Business Bureau of New York say that as a consumer of home care services you have the following rights:

- To receive considerate and respectful care in your home at all times;
- To participate in the development of your plan of care, including an explanation of any services proposed, and of alternative services that may be available in the community;
- To receive complete and written information on your plan of care, including the name of the supervisor responsible for your services;
- To refuse medical treatment or other services provided by law and to be informed of the possible results of your actions;
- To privacy and confidentiality about your health, social and financial circumstances, and what takes place in your home;
- To know that all communications and records will be treated confidentially;
- To expect that all home care personnel within the limits set by the plan of care will respond in good faith to your requests for assistance in the home;
- To receive information on an agency's policies and procedures including information on costs, qualifications of personnel, and supervision;
- To home care as long as needed and available;
- To examine all bills for service regardless of whether they are paid for out-of-pocket or through other sources of payment; and
- To receive nursing supervision of the paraprofessional if medically related personnel care is needed.

(From: *All About Home Care: A Consumer's Guide.* Courtesy of the National HomeCaring Council, Division of the Foundation for Hospice and Homecare)

formulates the plan of care, and performs skilled nursing procedures. The licensed practical nurse also gives skilled nursing care under the direction of the registered nurse. A home health aide gives personal care such as bathing and enemas. This person may also do some homemaking chores such as preparing a meal. A companion/sitter will sit with the patient and do routine household tasks. A sitter can be responsible only for simple needs that arise during the course of a visit, such as giving the patient a glass of water. Responsibilities at each level vary according to the needs of the individual patient and according to the care-giver's abilities. Agencies may have different titles for these personnel but the levels of care are similar.

Characteristics of Home Health Nursing

The home health care nurse must remain current on the family situation in the home, what has happened, what is new, what is changed. Days, weeks, or even a month can elapse between visits, making it necessary for data collection and assessment to include a review of past events. The interest the nurse shows in family members as individuals helps to establish a trusting relationship. Depending on the circumstances, the nurse confers with the other members of the home health care team at regular intervals.

A physician's order is a prerequisite for home care. Physician contact with homebound patients who have chronic conditions may be very limited, and telephone contact with the nurse is a primary source of data for that physician. A home health care nurse must be able to give accurate reports and make independent nursing decisions.

The patient and his family are in control in home health care. The situation is somewhat reversed from what it is in the hospital. That is, the nurse depends on the family for information in the home in much the same way that the family depends on the nurse in the hospital setting.

The home health care nurse must be comfortable coming and going in other people's homes and must do so in a nonjudgmental manner. What looks like unacceptable living conditions to a nurse may be a comfortable, safe environment to the older patient. A nurse's suggestions for improvement must be carefully made and made only from a standpoint of good health.

Many older people who use home health care have chronic, progressive conditions that are ultimately fatal, like cancer and Alzheimer's disease. The long-term goal is to permit these patients to stay in the home. Many of the problems they develop can not be solved by good nursing care, but these problems nevertheless must be managed so that they will not get worse. Assessment of the patient while giving bedside care and communication among the nursing team members are key factors in ongoing care (see the display, "A Preventive Home Health Nursing Plan").

Dying at home is once more becoming common. Some home health care patients prefer not to accept the various aspects of hospice care.

A Preventive Home Health Nursing Plan

Patient Situation:

C.H. is an 89-year-old female with Alzheimer's disease and is bedridden and totally dependent. She lives with her husband, who is 90 years old, and his 82-year-old brother. She receives personal care seven days a week by a home health licensed practical nurse. C.H. has a deep decubitus ulcer on her left hip and it is draining a serous fluid, sometimes blood-tinged. It will undoubtedly keep on draining until she dies. Other than that, her skin is in good condition. Her husband turns her several times during the night. She has flexion contractures of her arms, hips, and knees. A few years ago she suffered a stroke and, as a result, she has difficulty swallowing. Her tongue protrudes slightly. A suction machine is kept in the patient's bedroom for use by the L.P.N. if the patient chokes when she is being given fluids. Her husband patiently feeds her a liquid diet, with the head of her bed up about 45 degrees. Every day after C.H. has been bathed, the L.P.N. and C.H.'s husband get her into a wheelchair with the help of a Hoyer lift. Then she is wheeled into the living room where she sits for about an hour by the window with her husband. He talks to her and strokes her arm.

Patient Care Goals
1. Prevent
   - Infection in the decubitus ulcer
   - Urinary tract infection
   - Respiratory infection
   - Further skin breakdown
2. Keep patient comfortable
3. Provide adequate nourishment

Nursing Action	Rationale
1. Irrigate the decubitus ulcer with ½ strength hydrogen peroxide; note color of drainage and any odor. Pack with sterile gauze soaked in normal saline.	Keep ulcer clean to prevent infection. Greenish yellow drainage and odor are signs of infection.
2. Give complete bed bath. Apply dry powder in creased areas such as groin	Age and immobility increase the possibility of skin breakdown. Moist skin against

(continued)

A Preventive Home Health Nursing Plan *(Continued)*

Nursing Action	Rationale
and axillae, where skin touches skin. Rub back and extremities with lotion, and apply to bony prominences. Inspect skin closely.	skin will cause maceration. Rubbing increases circulation.
3. Patient has no teeth. Clean mouth and tongue with mild mouthwash and swabs. Observe for white patches.	White patches indicate candidiasis, a yeast infection. Debilitating disease and breakdown in the mucous membrane and the warm moist interior of the mouth create an ideal environment for this condition.
4. Note character of respirations.	Continuous noisy breathing may indicate a respiratory infection.
5. When cleansing the genital area, wash thoroughly around the catheter with soap and water and dry completely.	Cleanliness around the catheter will aid in preventing urinary tract infection.
6. Check for white thick vaginal drainage.	This is evidence of candidiasis (see number 3).
7. Measure 24-hour output— if less than 1000 ml, call R.N.	Patient may be going into renal failure.
8. Observe color and odor of urine.	Cloudy, foul-smelling, or bloody urine is a sign of urinary tract infection.
9. Take rectal temperature daily. If elevated over 100°F, notify R.N.	Elderly people can have a serious infection with only a minimal elevation of body temperature.
10. Give Fleets enema every other day.	This measure has kept the patient from becoming impacted with stool.

continued

A Preventive Home Health Nursing Plan *(Continued)*

Nursing Action	Rationale
11. Check alternating pressure mattress to be certain it is working.	Alternating pressure reduces the amount of pressure on any one point and helps prevent skin breakdown.
12. Put a small pillow between the patient's knees when she is back in bed.	Keeping the knees separated by a pillow prevents skin breakdown and further adduction hip contractures.
13. Take all extremities through range of motion.	This will prevent further contraction and increase circulation.

Note: All described signs of infection and other developments must be reported to the primary nurse as soon as possible.

These persons and their family members need to be gradually prepared for what will happen. However, the nurse can answer only questions that are asked. The older person may know he is going to die and, having acknowledged it once, will never seriously bring the subject up again. In cases in which the family has decided not to tell the older person about his prognosis, the nurse must respect that decision.

The deterioration of the loved one may be harder to deal with than his death. The family needs to be able to provide the care needed by the older loved one even though weakness makes all care more difficult. The nurse must anticipate both the patient's and the family's needs, for instance, in suggesting a bedside commode before it becomes a necessity. Fears should be identified and resolved. The daughter of a dying woman may say, "I am not afraid of mother's dying, but I'm scared stiff I'll do something wrong."

The nurse gets cues from family members when more information and support are needed. For instance, an elderly woman whose husband has cancer calls on the weekend to say that her husband is "different," perhaps sleeping 20 out of 24 hours and not taking medications. She asks what to do. During a home visit, the nurse tells the wife that the dying process has begun and gives her the written information on what to expect (see the display, "Signs of Approaching Death"). Helping family

Signs of Approaching Death and What to Do to Add Comfort

The Hospice staff understands and supports your desire to aid your loved one in dying in familiar surroundings. We also realize that this period of time may be a very difficult one for you and your family to live through. Because "fear of the unknown" is always greater than the "fear of the known," we want to be as open and honest with you as we possibly can. We give you this sheet of information to help you prepare for, anticipate, and understand symptoms that you may observe as your loved one approaches the final stages of life. *Not all these symptoms will appear at the same time, and may never appear.* Your Hospice staff is always available for information, support, and service.

1. You may notice your loved one having confusion about time, place, and identity of people. This is also a result of metabolic changes.
   Do: Remind your family member of the time, day, and who is with him/her.
2. Hearing and vision will lessen as the nervous system slows.
   Do: Keep lights on in the room. *NEVER* assume the patient cannot hear you. *ALWAYS* talk to him/her as if hearing were intact. Explain what you are doing; show your feelings.
3. The Hospice patient will tend to sleep more and more and may be difficult to awaken. This is a result of metabolic changes.
   Do: Plan activities and communicate at times when he/she seems more alert.
4. Your loved one will not take food or fluids as the need for these decreases.
   Do: Moisten mouth with a moist cloth. Clean oral cavity every ½ to 2 hours with wet Q-Tips. Keep lips wet with a lip balm.
5. There may be restlessness, pulling at bed linens, having visions you cannot see. This happens as a result of slowed circulation and less oxygen to the brain.
   Do: Stay calm, speak slowly and assuredly. Do not agree with inaccuracy to reality, but comfort with gentle reminders to time, place, and person.

(continued)

Signs of Approaching Death and What to Do to Add Comfort (Continued)

6. Loss of control of bowel and bladder may occur as death approaches, as the nervous system changes.
   Do: Ask the Hospice nurse for pads to place under the patient and for information on skin hygiene. Explore the possibility of a catheter for urine drainage.

7. If your loved one has a bladder catheter in place, you will notice a decreased amount of urine as kidney function slows.
   Do: You may need to irrigate the tube to prevent blockage. If you have not been taught to do this, contact a hospice nurse.

8. Arms and legs may become cool to touch and the underside of the body may become darker as circulation slows down.
   Do: Use warm blankets to protect the patient from feeling cold. Do not use electric blankets, since tissue integrity is changing and there is a danger of burns.

9. You may notice irregular breathing patterns and there may be spaces of time (10–30 seconds) of no breathing. This is a common symptom of decreased circulation.
   Do: Elevate the head by raising the bed or using pillows.

10. Due to a decrease in oral intake, your loved one may not be able to cough up secretions. These secretions may collect in the back of the throat causing noisy breathing. This has been referred to as the "death rattle."
    Do: Use a cool mist humidifier in the room. Elevate the head of the bed (if using a hospital bed) or add extra pillows. Ice chips (if the patient can swallow) or a cool, moist washcloth to the mouth can relieve feeling of thirst. Positioning on a side may help.

How Do You Know Death Has Occurred?

You will see this when death has occurred:

1. Pupils fixed and eyelids slightly opened in a stare.
2. No breathing.
3. No pulse.
4. No response to shaking or verbal stimulation.
5. Loss of bowel or bladder contents.
6. Relaxed jaw with mouth slightly open.

(continued)

Signs of Approaching Death and What to Do to Add Comfort (Continued)

What Do You Do When Death Has Occurred?

If you suspect your loved one has died, call the Hospice nurse. We are prepared to come to your home and help you at this time, 24 hours per day. It will not be necessary for you to call any other professional help. We will come to your home and help you with any other calls necessary. Please remember, help is always as close as your telephone, and we are dedicated to helping you and your loved one in this stressful time of change and grief. Please call us at any time you may have a question and we will do our best to help you help your loved one in any way possible.

(Courtesy of Bellin Hospital Hospice Program, Green Bay, Wisconsin.)

members one step at a time eases their way and allows the older person to die at home.

Written Forms

Each home health care agency has its own type of interview and assessment forms similar to those used by hospitals. There may be a short form, for example, for the postoperative patient who needs dressing changes until a family member learns how to do them. Long forms are more appropriate for the patient with a chronic disease. The difference in length of these forms will be due to the amount of physical assessment data that must be collected. An in-depth systems review is essential for a long-term patient. Every assessment form should include a "Life System Profile" (Fig. 10–4) and sections for data collection about support systems, other community resources needed, and emergency plans. The patient care plan may be written on a standard form and updated at regular intervals (Fig. 10–5).

Selecting a Nursing Home

In the future, it is likely that more older people will go directly from their own homes — rather than from a hospital — into nursing homes. In
(Text continues on p. 310.)

LIFE SYSTEM PROFILE:
Activities of Daily Living (Check appropriate boxes)

LEVEL OF INDEPENDENCE	WITHOUT HELP	USES A DEVICE	HELP OF ANOTHER	DEVICE & HELP	DEPENDENT/ DOES NOT DO	COMMENTS
Eating						
Toileting, Urinal Commode, Bathroom						
Transfers						
Walking						
Shopping, Cleaning, Laundry						
Bathing/Showering						
Dressing						
Meal Preparation						
Transportation						
Finances						

Figure 10–4. From a nursing assessment form. (Courtesy of Bellin Memorial Home Health Agency, Green Bay, Wisconsin)

NAME: LPN Assignment

TC = Total Care/ PC = Part Care/ SC = Self Care	TC	PC	SC	Special Instructions:
Bath-[ ] Tub [ ] Shower [ ] Bed				
Oral-[ ] Routine [ ] Dentures				
Hair-[ ] Comb/Brush [ ] Shampoo				
Shave				
Nails				
Dress				
Bladder-[ ] Cath. [ ] Incont.				
[ ] Foley Cath Care				
Bowel-[ ] Enema [ ] Involuntary				
[ ] Fleets Enema [ ] S.S. Enema				
[ ] Notify RN if no BM × 3 days				
Ostomy - type				
Ambulate				
Transfer				
Bed rest/Reposition				
ROM [ ] Active [ ] Passive				

Skin Care:

_____

Meals: Diet: _____
              [ ] Feed [ ] Assist [ ] Encourage Fluids

_____

Allergies:

_____

(continued)

Figure 10–5. Information form for a home health agency. (Courtesy of Bellin Memorial Hospital Home Health Agency, Green Bay, Wisconsin)

Special-Likes/Dislikes: _____

Impairments: [ ] Speech [ ] Hearing [ ] Vision [ ] Other_____

Mental Status: [ ] Oriented [ ] Forgetful [ ] Disoriented [ ] Comatose
             [ ] Depressed [ ] Lethargic [ ] Agitated [ ] Other_____

Medications: See med profile for scheduled meds. Specific instructions for use of PRN meds:

Special Instructions: Code [ ] No Code [ ]
(Vitals, treatments, safety concerns, etc)

Homemaking [ ] Clean Bathroom [ ] Dishes [ ] Laundry [ ] Meal Preparation
           [ ] Straighten and clean patient area for safety and general cleanliness.
           Special Instructions: _____

Primary R.N.   Date

(Fig. 10–5 continued)

selecting the right nursing home for a particular person, one should consider factors related to services provided, quality of care, environment, and cost. This can only be done by visiting facilities, asking specific questions, and making observations.

There will be times when the nurse is asked for advice in this matter. For example, when an apprehensive family takes an aging parent home from the hospital, a common question is, "I wonder how long it will be before I need to put her in a nursing home?" The nurse cannot give the answer, but in discussing this concern with the family member, the subject of what to look for in a nursing home can easily arise and the nurse should be prepared to suggest guidelines. Here is a list of possible questions to be answered in screening nursing homes:

- Is the nursing home licensed by the state, does it have a licensed administrator, and is it a member of a health care association such as the American Association of Homes for the Aging?

- Is it certified for Medicare and Medicaid reimbursement or is it a private-pay facility?
- Does the level of care meet the needs of the individual?
- Are the services and fees clearly stated?
- What happens if financial resources are depleted and this is a private-pay facility?
- Are the building and grounds in good condition?
- Are there places to walk or sit out-of-doors?
- Is the inside atmosphere pleasant and bright?
- Is the furniture comfortable?
- Are the rooms and bathrooms spacious and easy to move around in?
- What are the menus like, and does the dietary department consider individual preferences?
- What kind of staff is there, and what are their educational and training requirements?
- Are the social activities appealing?
- Is there any provision for transportation?
- What kind of contact is there with clergy, and are there scheduled religious services?
- Is there a "Resident's Bill of Rights?"

Under state and federal law, all nursing homes must have a bill of rights for residents that is prominently displayed and that has been interpreted to each resident or his designated guardian. These documents may vary in language, but they all recognize the same basic rights:

- To communicate privately with persons of one's choice
- To control one's own correspondence and receive mail unopened
- To have reasonable access to a telephone
- To remain in charge of decisions about personal financial affairs or designate another to do so
- To know the details of one's condition and treatment
- To choose one's own licensed, certified, or registered health care provider and pharmacist
- To have physical and emotional privacy
- To have adequate and appropriate care within the facility
- To have confidentiality
- To be treated with dignity and respect
- To be free from mental and physical abuse and from chemical and physical restraint except when authorized in writing by the physician for a specific time and purpose
- To remain in the facility and to be transferred or discharged only for designated reasons

- To have one's own religious and social activities
- To retain own possessions
- To have privacy with spouse
- To be free from discrimination or identification based on source of financial assistance
- To have a detailed explanation of services and charges and to be able to purchase those services needed regardless of sources of payment
- To exercise rights as a resident and citizen and to voice grievances

The rights of a nursing home resident can only be modified by authorization of the physician and the resident or resident's designated representative.

When a nursing home is finally selected, a visit to the older person's home by the social worker and a nurse might be arranged so that they can identify special needs. At this time, decisions can be made about what possessions can be transferred to the nursing home to make the individual's room more home-like.

Summary

Local resources for care of aging people depend on the size of the community. Churches and libraries can be starting points for the search when a community is small. On a state level, the Area Agency on Aging has a wealth of information. An assessment of needs will give one a general idea of where to look for help next. Some resources that make it possible for older people to live independently include transportation systems (often located through the American Red Cross), senior centers, and legal service agencies supported under the Older Americans Act and the Social Security Agency. Protective services, meal programs, medical equipment, counseling, and emergency assistance are available in many communities.

For older people who are more dependent, the appropriate resources may be rehabilitation services, adult day care centers, respite care, and residential care facilities. Home health care agencies help older people stay home even though they are ill, and in many cases this aids in recovery. For the patient who prefers to die at home, this kind of care is the answer. Home health offers the nurse an opportunity to work more independently than she would in a hospital. When selecting a nursing home, one should consider the services provided, quality of care, credentials of personnel, environment, and cost.

Activities

1. Report on one of the following in your community:
   a. The activities of a support group
   b. Medical equipment sources
   c. Transportation for senior citizens
   d. A program of activities for a senior center
   e. Availability of respite care
   f. Any other resource for elderly people
2. Interview a staff member from a home health care agency about the kinds of older people they see.
3. Describe in detail the features in a nursing home you would want for yourself, if you ever need to enter one. Also discuss what concerns you might have.
4. Suppose an older relative is suddenly confined to a wheelchair with a CVA and left-sided hemiplegia. Identify the arrangements that might have to be made so that he can live at home. Be specific.
5. With a specific older person in mind, visit and screen two nursing homes, using the questions in this chapter.

Bibliography

Auerbach M, Taylor M, Morosy J: Home care challenge: Care of the vulnerable elderly. Caring 4:38–40, 42, 1985

Birchenall J, Streight M: Care of the Older Adult, 2nd ed. Philadelphia, JB Lippincott, 1982

Burgess W: Community Health Nursing: Philosophy, Process, and Practice. Norwalk, CT, Appleton Century Crofts, 1983

Burnside I: Nursing and the Aged: A Self-Care Approach, 3rd ed. New York, McGraw-Hill, 1988

Christopher M: Home care for the elderly: In three-part harmony . . . assessment of the patient's health, home, and community. Nursing 16:50–55, 1986

Dychtwald K: Wellness and Health Promotion for the Elderly. Rockville, Aspen, 1986

Ebersole P, Hess P: Toward Healthy Aging: Human Needs and Nursing Response, 2nd ed. St. Louis, CV Mosby, 1985

Goto L, Braun K: Nursing home without walls . . . long-term care services in their homes. J Gerontol Nurs 13:6–9, 1987

Hall G: Care of the patient with Alzheimer's disease living at home. Nurs Clin North Am 23:31–45, 1988

Looney K: The respite care alternative. J Gerontol Nurs 13:18–21, 1987

Masson V: How nursing happens in adult day care. Geriatr Nurs 7:18–21, 1986

Portnow J, Houtmann M: Home Care for the Elderly: A Complete Guide. New York, McGraw-Hill, 1987

Pringle D: Humanistic care of the aged: The community perspective. Perspective 11:11–14, 1987

Quiring J: Helping the patient and family adjust to L.T.C. living. Nursing 16:60–63, 1986

Rosdahl C: Textbook of Basic Nursing, 4th ed. Philadelphia, JB Lippincott, 1985

Spradley B: Community Health Nursing: Concepts and Practice, 2nd ed. Boston, Little, Brown & Co, 1985

Walsh J, Persons C, Wieck L: Manual of Home Health Care Nursing. Philadelphia, JB Lippincott, 1987

Yurick A, Spier B, Robb S et al: The Aged Person and the Nursing Process, 2nd ed. Norwalk, CT, Appleton Century Crofts, 1984

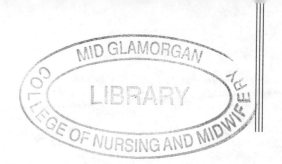

Index

Page numbers followed by *f* indicate figures; page numbers followed by *t* indicate tabular material.

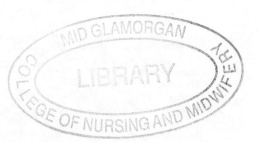